Dosage

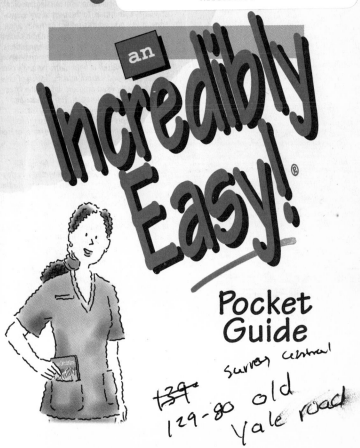

an

Incredibly
Easy! ®

Pocket
Guide

Surrey central
~~t39~~
129-80 old
Yale road

Lippincott Williams & Wilkins
a Wolters Kluwer business
Philadelphia · Baltimore · New York · London
Buenos Aires · Hong Kong · Sydney · Tokyo

back.
4 778-858-6576

Staff

Executive Publisher
Judith A. Schilling McCann, RN, MSN

Editorial Director
David Moreau

Clinical Director
Joan M. Robinson, RN, MSN

Art Director
Mary Ludwicki

Senior Managing Editor
Tracy S. Diehl

Clinical Project Manager
Jennifer Meyering, RN, BSN, MS, CCRN

Editors
Jo Donofrio, Diane Labus

Copy Editors
Kimberly Bilotta (supervisor), Scotti Cohn,
Amy Furman, Shana Harrington,
Dorothy P. Terry, Pamela Wingrod

Designer
Lynn Foulk

Illustrators
Bot Roda, Leah Rhoades Purvis

Digital Composition Services
Diane Paluba (manager), Joyce Rossi Biletz,
Donna S. Morris

Associate Manufacturing Manager
Beth J. Welsh

Editorial Assistants
Megan L. Aldinger, Karen J. Kirk,
Linda K. Ruhf

Design Assistant
Georg W. Purvis IV

Indexer
Karen C. Comerford

DCIEPG011106

Library of Congress Cataloging-in-Publication Data
Dosage calculations : an incredibly easy pocket guide.
    p. ; cm.
    Includes bibliographical references and index.
    1. Pharmaceutical arithmetic — Handbooks, manuals, etc. I. Lippincott Williams & Wilkins.
    [DNLM: 1. Pharmaceutical Preparations — administration & dosage — Handbooks. 2. Pharmaceutical Preparations — administration & dosage — Nurses' Instruction.
    3. Mathematics — Handbooks.
    4. Mathematics — Nurses' Instruction.
QV39 D722 2007]
RS57.D668 2007
615'.1401513 — dc22
ISBN-13: 978-1-58255-537-9
ISBN-10: 1-58255-537-0 (alk. paper)   2006025969

Contents

Contributors and consultants

Melody C. Antoon, RN, MSN
Instructor of Nursing
Lamar State College
Port Arthur, Tex.

Marissa R. K. Collins, BA
Consultant
Dresher, Pa.

Christine Frazer, RN, MSN, CNS
Nursing Instructor
Pennsylvania State University
Hershey

Julia A. Greenawalt, RNC, MA, MSN
Adjunct Faculty
University of Pittsburgh
School Nurse
Seneca Valley School District
Harmony, Pa.

Nancy Haynes, RN, MN, CCRN
Assistant Professor of Nursing
Saint Luke's College
Kansas City, Mo.

Patricia Lange-Otsuka, APRN, BC, MSN, EdD
Associate Professor of Nursing
Hawaii Pacific University
Kaneohe

Kathy Latch-Johnson, RN, MSN
Assistant Professor of Nursing
Baptist College of Health Sciences
Memphis

Linda May-Ludwig, RN, BS, MEd
Practical Nursing Instructor
Canadian Valley Technology Center
El Reno, Okla.

Catherine Todd Magel, RN, BC, EdD
Assistant Professor
Villanova (Pa.) University College of Nursing

Patricia O'Brien, RN, BS, MSN, APRN
Family Nurse Practitioner
Associate Professor, Graduate Nursing
Winona State University
Rochester, Minn.

Terri M. Perkins, RN, MSN
Instructor, Associate Degree Nursing
Program
Bellevue (Wash.) Community College

Dana Reeves, RN, MSN
Assistant Professor
University of Arkansas
Fort Smith

Allison Jones Terry, RN, MSN
Director of Community Certification
State of Alabama Department of Mental
Health and Mental Retardation
Montgomery

Karen Wilkinson, ARNP, MN
Nurse Practitioner, Pain Management
Program
Children's Hospital and Regional Medical
Center
Seattle

Sharon Wing, RN, MSN
Assistant Professor
Cleveland State University

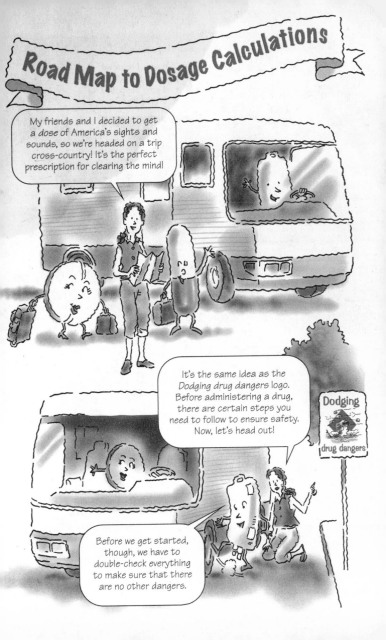

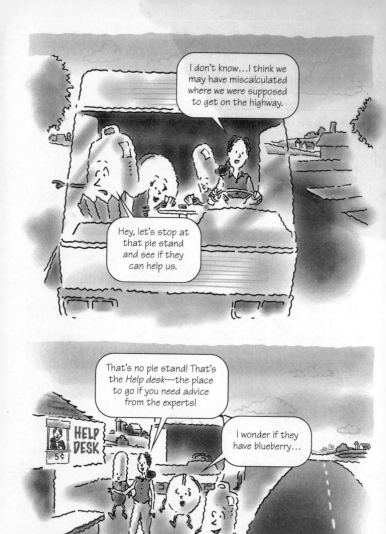

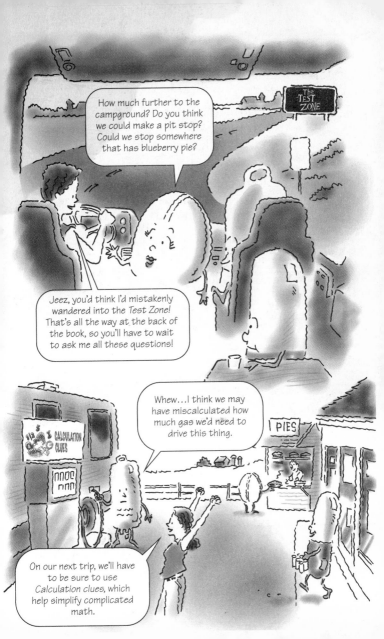

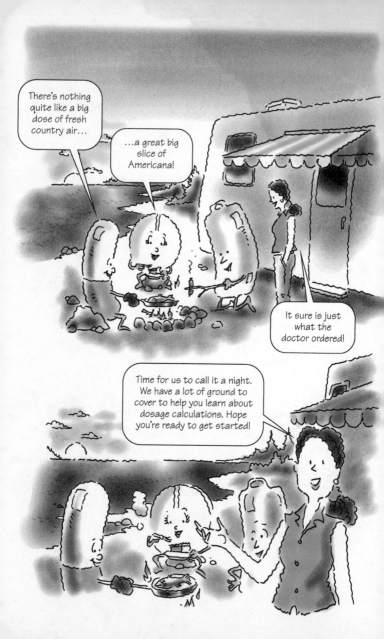

Math
basics

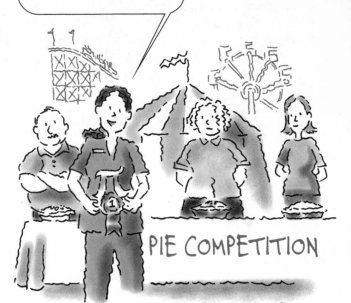

I'm so glad I read this chapter on fractions, decimals, percentages, conversions, and ratios and proportions before entering this "pi" competition.

PIE COMPETITION

A look at fractions

- A fraction represents the division of one number by another number; it's a mathematical expression for parts of a whole.
- The bottom number, the *denominator*, represents the total number of equal parts in the whole.
  – The larger the denominator, the greater the number of equal parts.
  – Another way of looking at it: As the denominator gets bigger, the size of each part will need to be smaller.

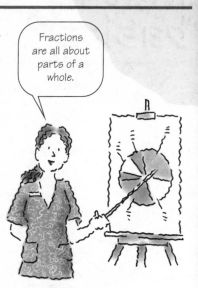

> Fractions are all about parts of a whole.

Parts of a whole

In any fraction, the numerator (top number) and the denominator (bottom number) represent the parts of a whole. The denominator describes the total number of equal parts in the whole; the numerator describes the number of parts being considered.

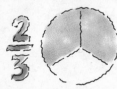

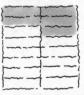

- The top number, the *numerator*, is the number of parts of the whole being considered.

Types of fractions

- Common: Both the numerator and denominator are whole numbers, such as $^2/_3$
- Complex: Both the numerator and denominator are fractions, such as $\dfrac{^2/_7}{^5/_{16}}$

- Proper: The numerator is smaller than the denominator, such as $^1/_4$
- Improper: The numerator is larger than the denominator, such as $^{11}/_4$
  – Will always represent a number that's greater than 1
  – Can also be written as a mixed number (a whole number and a fraction); for example, $^{11}/_4$ can be rewritten as $2^3/_4$

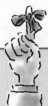

Memory jogger

To remember which number is the numerator and which is the denominator in a fraction, think of:

Nursing

Diagnosis.

The Numerator is on the top; the Denominator is on the bottom.

Working with fractions

- There are three ways to manipulate fractions:

  ☝ Convert mixed numbers to improper fractions and vice versa.

  ✌ Reduce fractions to their lowest terms.

  ✋ Find a common denominator.

> Changing fractions into different forms may seem like magic, but it's really pretty easy, as you'll see.

Converting mixed numbers and improper fractions

To convert a mixed number to an improper fraction

- Multiply the denominator by the whole number.
- Add the product, or resulting number, from the first step to the numerator (you'll get a new numerator).
- Leave the denominator as is.

To convert an improper fraction back to a mixed number

- Divide the numerator by the denominator; the result will be a whole number with something left over.
- Place the leftover number (the new numerator) over the old denominator.

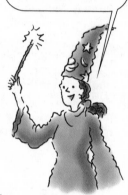

Learn by example

Convert $5\frac{1}{3}$ to an improper fraction.

- Multiply the denominator 3 by the whole number 5, for a total of 15.
- Add 15 to the numerator 1, for a new numerator of 16.
- Leave the denominator as is.
- The improper fraction is $\frac{16}{3}$.

Now convert $\frac{16}{3}$ back to a mixed number.

- Divide the numerator 16 by the denominator 3; you get 5 with 1 left over.
- The 1 becomes the new numerator, and the denominator stays the same.
- The mixed number is $5\frac{1}{3}$.

Reducing fractions to their lowest terms

- Fractions are usually reduced to their lowest terms, or the smallest numbers possible in the numerator and denominator.
- Reducing fractions is a two-step process:

    Determine the largest common divisor of the numerator and denominator (this is the largest number that both can be divided by).

    Divide the numerator and denominator by that number.

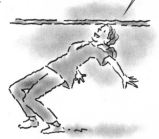

Remember with fractions, as in limbo, it's usually how low can you go?!

Learn by example

Reduce $^8/_{10}$ to its lowest terms.

- First, find the largest common divisor of 8 and 10, which is 2.
- Now divide the numerator and denominator by 2 to reduce the fraction to its lowest terms, or $^4/_5$.

$$\frac{8}{10} \text{ is } \frac{8 \div 2}{10 \div 2} \text{ is } \frac{4}{5}$$

Finding a common denominator

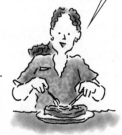

This prime rib is only divisible by 3—me, myself, and I.

- A common denominator is a multiple that all the denominators in a set of fractions share in common.
- One easy way to find a common denominator is to multiply all the denominators. For example, to find a common denominator for the fractions $^2/_5$ and $^7/_{10}$, multiply 5 and 10 to get the multiplied common denominator 50.
- The lowest common denominator is the smallest number that's a multiple of all the denominators in a set of fractions.
- One way to find the lowest common denominator for a set of fractions is to work with its prime factors.
  – A prime number is a number that's evenly divisible only by itself and 1.
  – Prime factors are prime numbers that can be divided into the denominators in a set of fractions.
- One method of finding the lowest common denominator is prime factoring, which uses a table format.

Learn by example

Find the lowest common denominator for ⅛, ¼, and ⅕.

- First, create a table with two headings: "Prime factors" and "Denominators."
- Write the denominators 8, 4, and 5 across the top right columns.

Prime factors	Denominators		
	8	4	5

- Divide the three denominators by the prime factors for each, starting with the smallest prime factor by which one of the denominators can be divided—in this case 2.
- Write 2 in the left-hand column, and divide the denominators by it.
- Bring down the numbers in the right-side columns that aren't evenly divisible by the prime factor in the left column—in this case the denominator 5 isn't divisible by the prime factor 2, so just bring the 5 down.

Prime factors	Denominators		
	÷ ←	8	4	5
2	=	4	2	5

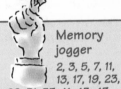

Memory
jogger

2, 3, 5, 7, 11,
13, 17, 19, 23,
29, 31, 37, 41, 43, 47,
53, 59, 61, 67, 71, 73,
79, 83, 89, 97

What do all these numbers have in common? They're all the prime numbers between 2 and 100. Remember, a prime number can only be divided by itself and 1.

- Repeat this process until the numbers in the bottom row can't be divided further.

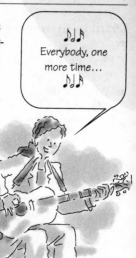

♪♪♪
Everybody, one
more time...
♪♪♪

Prime factors	Denominators		
	8	4	5
2	4	2	5
2	2	1	5
2	1	1	5

- Then multiply the prime factors in the left column by the numbers in the bottom row.

$$2 \times 2 \times 2 \times 1 \times 1 \times 5 = 40$$

The lowest common denominator for this set of fractions is 40.

Converting a set of fractions

- When you know the lowest common denominator of a set of fractions, you can convert the fractions so they'll all have the same denominator—the lowest common denominator.

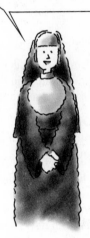

Did I just hear correctly...they're **all** converting? Oh how heavenly!

Multiplying by 1 in the form of a fraction

- One way to convert a set of fractions is to multiply each fraction by 1 in the form of a fraction—that is, a fraction with the same number in the numerator and denominator.
- You can find this fraction by taking the lowest common denominator and dividing it by the original denominator.

$$\frac{\text{original}}{\text{fraction}} \times \frac{\text{lowest common denominator} \div \text{original denominator}}{\text{lowest common denominator} \div \text{original denominator}}$$

Learn by example

Convert ⅛, ¼, and ⅕ so that each has the lowest common denominator.

- We already know that the lowest common denominator for this set of fractions is 40.
- Here's the conversion of the first fraction, ⅛, to ⁵⁄₄₀:

$$\frac{1}{8} = \frac{1}{8} \times \frac{40 \div 8}{40 \div 8} = \frac{1}{8} \times \frac{5}{5} = \frac{1 \times 5}{8 \times 5} = \frac{5}{40}$$

- Convert the next fraction, ¼, to ¹⁰⁄₄₀:

$$\frac{1}{4} = \frac{1}{4} \times \frac{40 \div 4}{40 \div 4} = \frac{1}{4} \times \frac{10}{10} = \frac{1 \times 10}{4 \times 10} = \frac{10}{40}$$

- Convert the last fraction in the set, ⅕, to ⁸⁄₄₀:

$$\frac{1}{5} = \frac{1}{5} \times \frac{40 \div 5}{40 \div 5} = \frac{1}{5} \times \frac{8}{8} = \frac{1 \times 8}{5 \times 8} = \frac{8}{40}$$

Using long division

- You can also convert a set of fractions using long division following these steps:

    ☝ Divide the lowest common denominator by the original denominator.

    ✌ Multiply the quotient (the resulting number) by the original numerator to determine the new numerator.

    🤟 Place the new numerator over the lowest common denominator.

- Here's the conversion for each fraction:

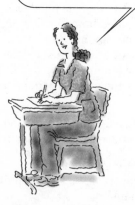

Long division...that really takes me back to my schoolgirl days! Now where did I leave my lunchbox?

$$\overset{\text{quotient}}{\underset{\text{original}}{\text{denominator}} \big) \overset{}{\underset{\substack{\text{lowest} \\ \text{common} \\ \text{denominator}}}{}}} \times \overset{\text{original}}{\underset{\text{numerator}}{}} = \frac{\text{new numerator}}{\substack{\text{lowest} \\ \text{common} \\ \text{numerator}}}$$

Learn by example

Convert $\frac{3}{8}$, $\frac{1}{4}$, and $\frac{2}{5}$.

- We already know that the lowest common denominator is 40.
- Convert the first fraction in the set, $\frac{3}{8}$, to $\frac{15}{40}$:

$$\frac{3}{8} = \frac{5}{8\overline{)40}} \times 3 = \frac{15}{40}$$

- Next, convert $\frac{1}{4}$ to $\frac{10}{40}$:

$$\frac{1}{4} = \frac{10}{4\overline{)40}} \times 1 = \frac{10}{40}$$

- Now convert $\frac{2}{5}$ to $\frac{16}{40}$:

$$\frac{2}{5} = \frac{8}{5\overline{)40}} \times 2 = \frac{16}{40}$$

Comparing the relative size of fractions

- Finding the lowest common denominator in a set of fractions allows you to compare the relative size of fractions; this is especially useful when comparing strengths of medications.
- When comparing fractions with common denominators, the fraction with the largest numerator is always the largest number.

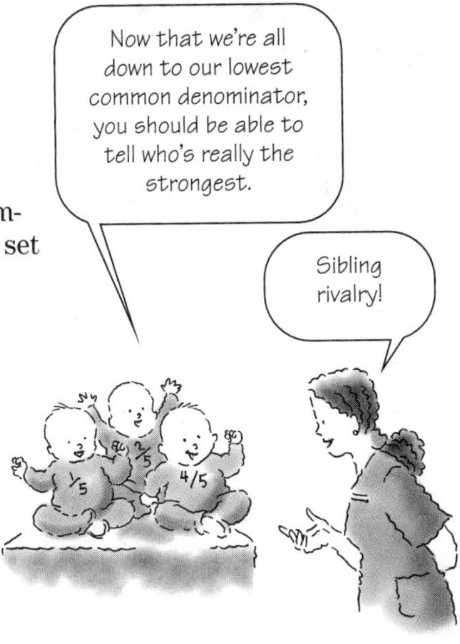
Now that we're all down to our lowest common denominator, you should be able to tell who's really the strongest.
Sibling rivalry!
1/5
2/5
4/5

Calculation clues

Denominators can be deceptive

If you were hungry, would you rather have 1 slice from a pie that was cut into 4 slices, 8 slices, or 16 slices? You'd choose 4, of course, because the slices would be bigger. You can judge the size of fractions the same way. When the fractions all have the same numerators—in this case, $\frac{1}{4}$, $\frac{1}{8}$, and $\frac{1}{16}$—the fraction with the lowest denominator is the biggest one. Don't fall into the trap of thinking that the bigger the denominator, the bigger the fraction. Think in terms of a pie, as shown here.

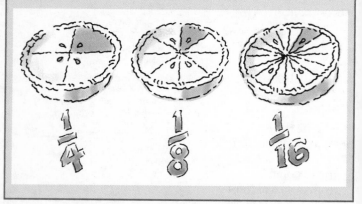

- Conversely, when comparing fractions with common numerators, the fraction with the lowest denominator is the largest number.

Learn by example: Converting with primes and 1 (in the form of a fraction)

Compare the strengths of sublingual nitroglycerin tablets.
- Tablets are available in $\frac{1}{100}$ grain, $\frac{1}{150}$ grain, and $\frac{1}{200}$ grain strengths.

- Using the prime factor method, first find the lowest common denominator for these three fractions.

Prime factors	Denominators		
	100	150	200
2	50	75	100
2	25	75	50
5	5	15	10
5	1	3	2

- Multiply the prime factors in the left column and the numbers in the bottom row:
$$2 \times 2 \times 5 \times 5 \times 1 \times 3 \times 2 = 600$$

- Next, convert all three fractions—$1/100$, $1/150$, and $1/200$—to new fractions with the lowest common denominator of 600. Multiply each fraction by 1 (in the form of a fraction) so that $1/100$ is converted to $6/600$:

$$\frac{1}{100} = \frac{1}{100} \times \frac{600 \div 100}{600 \div 100} = \frac{1}{100} \times \frac{6}{6} = \frac{1 \times 6}{100 \times 6} = \frac{6}{600}$$

and $1/150$ is converted to $4/600$:

$$\frac{1}{150} = \frac{1}{150} \times \frac{600 \div 150}{600 \div 150} = \frac{1}{150} \times \frac{4}{4} = \frac{1 \times 4}{150 \times 4} = \frac{4}{600}$$

and $1/200$ is converted to $3/600$:

$$\frac{1}{200} = \frac{1}{200} \times \frac{600 \div 200}{600 \div 200} = \frac{1}{200} \times \frac{3}{3} = \frac{1 \times 3}{200 \times 3} = \frac{3}{600}$$

- Now compare the final three fractions and you'll see that the $1/100$-grain nitroglycerin tablet offers the largest dose: $6/600$.

Learn by example: Converting with long division

You can also arrive at the same conclusion by dividing the lowest common denominator (600) by the denominator, multiplying the numerator by the number obtained, and placing the result over the lowest common denominator.

- $\frac{1}{100}$ is converted to $\frac{6}{600}$ this way:

$$\frac{1}{100} = \frac{6}{100\overline{)600}} \times 1 = \frac{6}{600}$$

- $\frac{1}{150}$ is converted to $\frac{4}{600}$ this way:

$$\frac{1}{150} = \frac{4}{150\overline{)600}} \times 1 = \frac{4}{600}$$

- $\frac{1}{200}$ is converted to $\frac{3}{600}$ this way:

$$\frac{1}{200} = \frac{3}{200\overline{)600}} \times 1 = \frac{3}{600}$$

Explore your alternatives...you'll discover that, even by a longer route, you'll arrive at the same conclusion.

Adding fractions

- To add fractions, first convert them to fractions with common denominators.
- Follow these three steps to add fractions:

    Find the lowest common denominator.

    Convert the fractions by multiplying by 1 (in the form of a fraction) to yield fractions with the lowest common denominator.

    Add the new fractions. To add fractions with a common denominator, add the numerators and place the result over the common denominator; the resulting fraction is your answer. (Remember to always reduce your answer to the lowest terms, if possible.)

Comparing apples to apples

When adding or subtracting fractions, don't forget to convert them to fractions with common denominators. That way, you'll be comparing apples to apples.

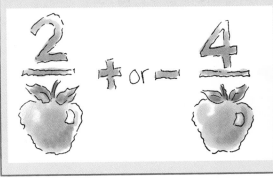

Learn by example

Add ½ and ⅕.

- Find the lowest common denominator. In this case, because the denominators 2 and 5 are both prime numbers, multiply 2 and 5 to find the lowest common denominator, 10.
- Convert the fractions by multiplying each by 1 (in the form of a fraction) to yield fractions with the lowest common denominator.
- Convert ½ to ⁵⁄₁₀:

$$\frac{1}{2} = \frac{1}{2} \times \frac{10 \div 2}{10 \div 2} = \frac{1}{2} \times \frac{5}{5} = \frac{1 \times 5}{2 \times 5} = \frac{5}{10}$$

- Next, convert ⅕ to ²⁄₁₀:

$$\frac{1}{5} = \frac{1}{5} \times \frac{10 \div 5}{10 \div 5} = \frac{1}{5} \times \frac{2}{2} = \frac{1 \times 2}{5 \times 2} = \frac{2}{10}$$

- Now add the converted fractions:

$$\frac{5}{10} + \frac{2}{10} = \frac{5+2}{10} = \frac{7}{10}$$

Adding fractions is as easy as 1, 2, 3!

Subtracting fractions

- To subtract fractions, first convert them to terms with common denominators.
- Then follow the same steps as for adding fractions, but use subtraction instead.

> This is always my favorite part—demonstrating the correct way to subtract one generous piece of pie from the whole. I just love my job!

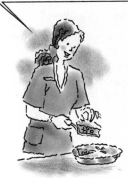

Learn by example

Subtract $\frac{1}{9}$ from $\frac{5}{6}$.

- Find the lowest common denominator—in this case, 18.
- Convert the fractions to those with the lowest common denominator by multiplying each fraction by the number 1 (in the form of a fraction).
- Convert $\frac{5}{6}$ to $\frac{15}{18}$:

$$\frac{5}{6} = \frac{5}{6} \times \frac{18 \div 6}{18 \div 6} = \frac{5}{6} \times \frac{3}{3} = \frac{5 \times 3}{6 \times 3} = \frac{15}{18}$$

- Then convert $\frac{1}{9}$ to $\frac{2}{18}$:

$$\frac{1}{9} = \frac{1}{9} \times \frac{18 \div 9}{18 \div 9} = \frac{1}{9} \times \frac{2}{2} = \frac{1 \times 2}{9 \times 2} = \frac{2}{18}$$

- Now subtract the numerators, and place the results over the common denominator. Reduce the fraction to its lowest terms, if possible. (In this case, the fraction can't be reduced.)

$$\frac{15}{18} - \frac{2}{18} = \frac{15 - 2}{18} = \frac{13}{18}$$

Multiplying fractions

- You don't need to convert to a common denominator when multiplying fractions.
- Simply multiply the numerators and denominators in turn to find the product.

Learn by example

Multiply ⁴⁄₇ by ⁵⁄₈.
- Set up the equation:

$$\frac{4}{7} \times \frac{5}{8}$$

- Multiple the numerators and multiply the denominators:

$$\frac{4 \times 5}{7 \times 8} = \frac{20}{56}$$

- Reduce the answer to its lowest terms:

$$\frac{5}{14}$$

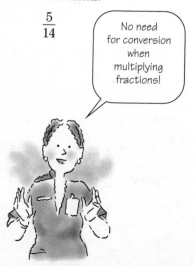

No need for conversion when multiplying fractions!

Dividing fractions

- Division problems are usually written as two fractions separated by a division sign.
  – The first fraction is the number to be divided (the dividend).
  – The second fraction is the number doing the dividing (the divisor).
  – The answer is the quotient.
- You don't need to convert to a common denominator when dividing fractions.
- You do need to invert (flip) the divisor and multiply the reciprocal by the dividend to complete the calculation.

Divvying up the problem

Before you can divide numbers, you need to know what each part of a division problem is called. This division problem can be written two different ways, but the terms remain the same.

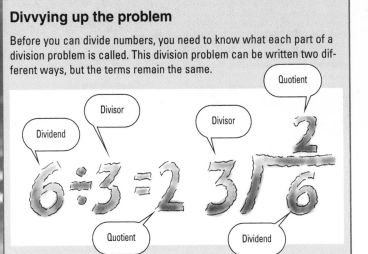

Dividing simple fractions

- To divide fractions, first multiply the dividend by the divisor's reciprocal (inverted divisor).

- Then complete the calculation and reduce the answer (the quotient) to its lowest terms.

Learn by example
Divide $\frac{5}{7}$ by $\frac{2}{3}$.
- First, set up the problem:

$$\frac{5}{7} \div \frac{2}{3}$$

- Next, multiply the dividend by the divisor's reciprocal (inverted divisor):

$$\frac{5}{7} \div \frac{2}{3} = \frac{5}{7} \times \frac{3}{2}$$

- Complete the calculation, and reduce the answer (quotient) to its lowest terms:

$$\frac{5 \times 3}{7 \times 2} = \frac{15}{14} = 1\frac{1}{14}$$

Dividing by a whole number
- To divide a fraction by a whole number, follow the same principle as with simple fractions.
- To convert a whole number to a fraction, simply put the number over 1.

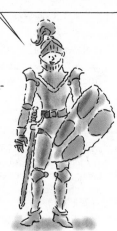

You mean there's no real dividing and conquering in a fraction division problem—just multiplying? Oh...how embarrassing!

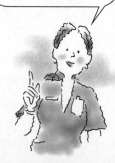

The number 1 is key when it comes to converting whole numbers to fractions.

Learn by example

Divide $\frac{3}{5}$ by 2.

- First, convert the whole number 2 to the fraction $\frac{2}{1}$:

$$\frac{3}{5} \div 2 = \frac{3}{5} \div \frac{2}{1}$$

- Then multiply the dividend ($\frac{3}{5}$) by the reciprocal of the divisor ($\frac{1}{2}$). Reduce the answer to its lowest terms:

$$\frac{3}{5} \times \frac{1}{2} = \frac{3 \times 1}{5 \times 2} = \frac{3}{10}$$

Dividing complex fractions

- In complex fractions, the numerators and denominators are fractions.
- They can be simplified by following the rules for division of fractions.

Learn by example

Divide $\frac{1}{3}$ by $\frac{5}{8}$.

- First, rewrite the complex fraction as a division problem:

$$\frac{\frac{1}{3}}{\frac{5}{8}} = \frac{1}{3} \div \frac{5}{8}$$

See, even dividing complex fractions is easy when you break it down into steps.

- Multiply the dividend ($\frac{1}{3}$) by the reciprocal of the divisor ($\frac{8}{5}$):

$$\frac{1}{3} \times \frac{8}{5}$$

- Last, complete the calculation:

$$\frac{1 \times 8}{3 \times 5} = \frac{8}{15}$$

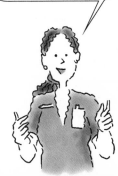

Deciphering decimals

- A decimal fraction is a proper fraction in which the denominator is a power of 10, signified by a decimal point placed at the left of the numerator; for example, 0.2 is the same as ²⁄₁₀.

- In a decimal number—for instance, 2.25—the decimal point separates the whole number from the decimal fraction.

- Each number or place to the left of the decimal point represents a whole number that's a power of 10.

- Each place to the right of the decimal point signifies a fraction whose denominator is a power of 10.

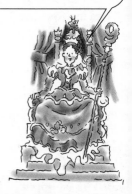

> I hate to admit it, but the decimal point holds all the real power around here—the power of 10 to be precise!

Know your places

Based on its position relative to the decimal point, each decimal place represents a power of 10 or a fraction with a denominator that's a power of 10, as shown below.

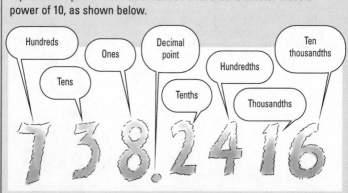

- When referring to decimal numbers in dosage calculations, use the term *point* to signify the decimal point.
- After performing mathematical functions with decimal numbers, you may eliminate zeros to the *right* of the decimal point that don't appear before other numbers.
- You may add zeros at the end of fractions for placeholders in calculations; deleting or adding zeros at the end of decimal fractions doesn't change the value of the number.
- When writing answers to mathematical calculations and specifying drug dosages, always put a zero to the *left* of the decimal point if no other number appears there; this helps prevent errors.

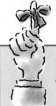

Memory jogger

To remember which zeros you can safely eliminate in a decimal number, think of the letters "l" and "r" in the words "left" and "right."

- **Leave** a zero to the **left** of the decimal point if no other number appears there and you need a placeholder (as in 0.5 ml).

- **Remove** any trailing zeros to the **right** of the decimal point if no other number follows and you don't need a placeholder (as in 7.50 mg).

Zap those zeros

Are you solving a problem with decimal numbers? In most cases, you can delete all zeros to the right of the decimal point that don't appear before other numbers.

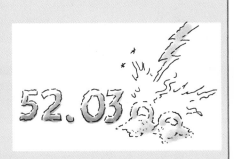

Adding and subtracting decimal fractions

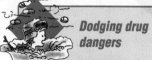

- Before adding and subtracting decimal fractions, align the decimal points vertically to help keep track of the decimal points.
- To maintain column alignment, add zeros as placeholders in decimal fractions.

Learn by example

Add 2.61, 0.315, and 4.8.

- To maintain column alignment, use zeros to align the decimals before adding the numbers:

```
  2.610
  0.315
+ 4.800
-------
  7.725
```

- Subtract 0.05 from 4.726.

```
  4.726
- 0.050
-------
  4.676
```

> Think of it this way—if you aren't careful, one little misplaced decimal point can wreak havoc with your checking account.

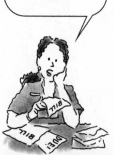

Disappearing decimal alert

Decimal points and zeros may be small items, but they're big deals on medication order sheets and administration records. When you get a drug order, study it closely. If a dose doesn't sound right, maybe a decimal point was left out or placed incorrectly.

For instance, an order that calls for ".5 mg lorazepam I.V." may be mistaken for "5 mg of lorazepam I.V." The correct way to write this order is to use a zero as a placeholder before the decimal point. The order would then become "0.5 mg lorazepam I.V."

Multiplying decimal fractions

- You don't need to align decimal points before multiplying decimal fractions.
- To determine where to place the decimal point in the final product, first add together the number of decimal places in both factors being multiplied.
- Then count out the same total number of places in the answer, starting from the right and moving to the left, and place the decimal point just to the left of the last place count.

Learn by example

Multiply 2.7 by 0.81.

$$
\begin{array}{r}
2.70 \\
\times\,0.81 \\
\hline
2.1870
\end{array}
$$

> Diving requires aligning yourself with the board. Dividing requires aligning those decimal points.

- In this case, the decimal point is placed after the 2 because there are four decimal places in the combined factors (notice the addition of a zero as a placeholder in the first factor).

Dividing decimal fractions

- When dividing decimal fractions, align the decimal points but don't add zeros as placeholders.
- Decimal point placement is easiest when the divisor is a whole number.

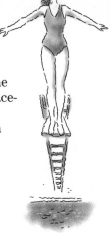

Calculation clues

Dividing decimal fractions

When dividing one decimal fraction by another, move the divisor's decimal point all the way to the right to convert it to a whole number. Move the dividend's decimal point the same number of places to the right. After completing the division problem, place the quotient's decimal point directly above the new decimal point in the dividend.

This example shows how to divide 10.45 by 2.6. The quotient is rounded to the nearest hundredth.

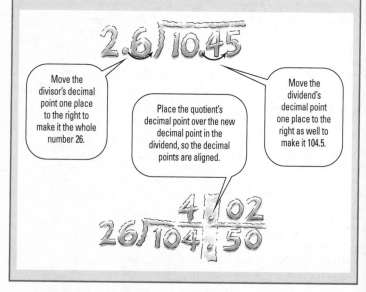

Move the divisor's decimal point one place to the right to make it the whole number 26.

Place the quotient's decimal point over the new decimal point in the dividend, so the decimal points are aligned.

Move the dividend's decimal point one place to the right as well to make it 104.5.

- Place the decimal point in the quotient directly above the decimal point in the dividend, and then work the problem.
- If the divisor is a decimal fraction, the decimal points in both the divisor and the dividend must be moved.

Learn by example

Divide 4.68 by 2.

$$2.34$$
$$2\overline{)4.68}$$

Rounding off decimal fractions

- In most nursing situations, you'll only need measurements to the tenth or hundredth place.
- If a decimal fraction is longer, you'll need to round it off—that is, convert the long fraction to one with fewer decimal places.

The round-off: A three-step maneuver

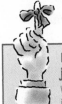

First, decide how many places to the right of the decimal point you want to keep. If you decide to round off the number to hundredths, keep two places to the right of the decimal point and delete the rest.

Second, look at the first deleted number to determine whether to round off. If the deleted number is 5 or greater, add 1 to the number in the hundredths place. If it's less than 5, leave the number as is.

Last, round off the decimal fraction accordingly.

Memory jogger

When rounding, remember that 5 is the magic number. Check the number to the right of the decimal place that will be rounded off. If that number is 5 or greater, then add 1 to the place. If it's less than 5, leave the number alone.

For example, try rounding off these numbers to the nearest hundredths:

- 6.447
- 2.992
- 4.119

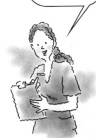

The answers are 6.45, 2.99, and 4.12.

Learn by example

Round off 14.723 to the nearest hundredth.

- First, determine which number is the hundredths place (2) and delete all the numbers to the right of it (in this case, the number 3).
- Because 3 is lower than 5, you don't add 1 to the 2.
- The rounded number is 14.72.

Converting decimal fractions

- Many measuring devices have metric calibrations, so you'll need to convert common (proper or mixed) fractions to decimal fractions and vice versa.
- To change a common (proper) fraction into a decimal fraction:
  - First, divide the numerator by the denominator.
  - Then add a zero as a placeholder to the left of the decimal point:

$$\tfrac{4}{10} = 4 \div 10 = 10\overline{)4.0}^{\,0.4}$$

- To convert a mixed number to a decimal fraction:
  - First, convert it to an improper fraction.
  - Then divide the numerator by the denominator:

$$4\tfrac{3}{4} = \frac{19}{4} = 19 \div 4 = 4\overline{)19.00}^{\,4.75}$$

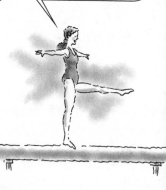

Working with fractions is kind of like gymnastics—you get to practice flips and round-offs but always need to keep in proper alignment.

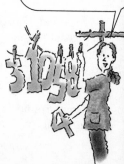

On Mondays, everything—even my numbers—needs changing and laundering.

- To convert a decimal fraction back to a common fraction:
  - Count the number of decimal places in the decimal fraction (this is the number of zeros in the denominator of the common fraction). For example, 0.33 has two decimal places, so the denominator of its common fraction is 100.
  - Remove the decimal point from 0.33, and use this number as the numerator. Reduce the fraction if possible.

$$0.33 = \frac{33}{100}$$

- To convert a decimal fraction back to a mixed number, use the same method previously described:

$$5.75 = \frac{575}{100} = 5^{75}/_{100} = 5\frac{3}{4}$$

Understanding percentages

- Percentages are another way to express fractions and numerical relationships.
- The percent symbol (%) can be used with whole numbers, mixed numbers, and decimals.

Converting percentages to decimals

- To change a percentage to a decimal fraction, remove the % sign and multiply the number in the percentage by $1/100$, or 0.01.

    $$84\% = 84 \times 0.01 = 0.84$$

- Be sure to shift the decimal point to the left when converting a percentage to a decimal.

Converting percentages to common fractions

- First, remove the percentage sign and put the decimal place two places to the left.
- Next, convert the decimal fraction to a common fraction with a denominator that's a factor of 10.
- Last, reduce the fraction to its lowest terms.

> **A point about percents**
>
> When you see %, the percent sign, think "for every hundred." Why? Because percentage means any quantity stated as parts per hundred. In other words, 75% is actually $75/100$ because the percent sign takes the place of the denominator 100.

> I wonder what percentage of my day is spent converting fractions to decimals and decimals to percentages?

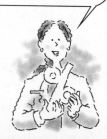

Calculation clues

From percentages to decimals (and back again)

Although it seems like a harmless dot, a misplaced decimal point can lead to a serious drug error. Study the examples below to see how to perform conversions quickly and accurately.

Jump to the left
To convert from a percentage to a decimal, remove the percent sign and move the decimal point two places to the *left*. Here's how:

$$97\% = 0.97$$

Jump to the right
To convert a decimal to a percentage, reverse the process. Move the decimal point two places to the *right,* add a zero as a placeholder if necessary, and then add a percent sign. If the resulting percentage is a whole number, remove the decimal because it's understood. Here's what the calculation looks like:

$$0.20 = 20\%$$

Learn by example

Convert 32.7% to a common fraction.

- First, remove the percentage sign and put the decimal point two places to the left, creating the decimal fraction 0.327.
- Then convert 0.327 to a common fraction using 1,000 as the denominator, because 0.327 has three decimal places:

$$32.7\% = 0.327 = {}^{327}/_{1,000}$$

- No need to reduce; this is already reduced to its lowest terms.

Converting common fractions to percentages

- First, create a decimal fraction by dividing the numerator by the denominator.
- Then convert the decimal fraction to a percentage by moving the decimal point two places to the right and adding the percent sign.

Learn by example

Convert ⅓ to a percentage.

- First, create a decimal fraction by dividing 1 by 3, rounding off the quotient to two decimal places:

$$\tfrac{1}{3} = 1 \div 3 = 0.333 = 0.33$$

- Then convert the decimal fraction to a percentage by moving the decimal point two places to the right and adding the percent sign:

$$0.33 = 33\%$$

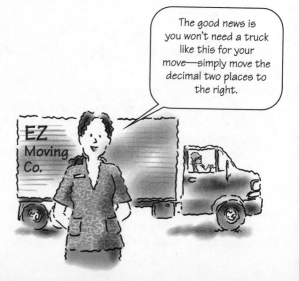

The good news is you won't need a truck like this for your move—simply move the decimal two places to the right.

Solving percentage problems

Three types of calculations may be used. They involve:

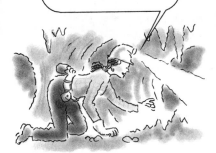 finding the percentage of a number

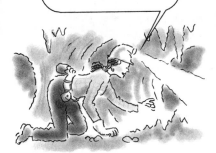 finding what percentage one number is of another

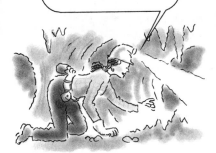 finding a number when a percentage of it is known.

> I'm not sure whether I'm looking for the percentage of a number or the number of a percentage, but I'm sure I'll know it when I find it.

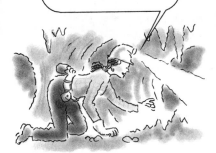

> ### Percentage problems: Watch the wording
>
> When a percentage problem is worded as: "What's 25% of 80?" mentally change the *of* to a multiplication sign so the problem becomes "What's 25% (or, using a decimal fraction, .25) × 80?" Then continue with the calculation. (The answer is 20.)
>   If a problem is worded as "25 is what percentage of 80?" treat the *what* as a division sign so the problem becomes $25/80$. Then continue with the calculation. (The answer is 0.3125, or 31.25%.)

Finding a percentage of a number

The question "What's 40% of 200?" is an example of this type of calculation. To solve the problem, follow these steps:

• First, change the word *of* to a multiplication sign:

$$40\% \times 200 = ?$$

- Next, convert 40% to a decimal fraction by removing the percentage sign and moving the decimal point two places to the left:

$$40\% = 0.40$$

- Then multiply the two numbers to get the answer (80).

$$0.40 \times 200 = 80$$

Learn by example

What's 5% of 150?
- First, restate as a multiplication problem:

$$5\% \times 150 = ?$$

- Next, convert 5% to a decimal fraction:

$$5\% = 0.05$$

- Now multiply the two numbers to get the answer:

$$0.05 \times 150 = 7.5$$

Finding what percentage one number is of another

- When you need to figure out what percentage one number is of another, set up your question as something like: "10 is what percentage of 200?" (The question may also be stated as "What percentage of 200 is 10?") To solve it, follow these steps:
  – First, restate the question as a division problem, with the number 10 as the dividend and the number 200 as the divisor:

$$\begin{array}{r} 0.05 \\ 200\overline{)10.00} \end{array}$$

– Then move the decimal point in the quotient two places to the right and add a percentage sign:

$$0.05 = 5\%$$

What to do with the remainder

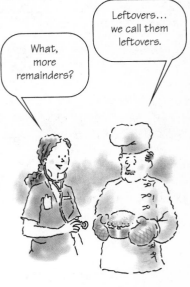

Leftovers... we call them leftovers.

What, more remainders?

• If the divisor doesn't divide exactly into the dividend, state the quotient as a decimal rounded to the nearest tenth. For example, "3 is what percentage of 11?"

– Restate the question as a division problem, making 11 the divisor and 3 the dividend. Work out the quotient to four places:

```
        0.2727
  11 ) 3.0000
        2 2
        ─────
          80
          77
        ─────
          30
          22
        ─────
          80
          77
        ─────
           3
```

– Move the decimal point two places to the right, and round to the nearest tenth:

$$0.2727 = 27.3\%$$

Learn by example

Determine that 5 is what percent of 22?

- Restate the question as a division problem, working to four places after the decimal:

$$
\begin{array}{r}
0.2272 \\
22\overline{)5.0000} \\
4\,4 \\
\hline
60 \\
44 \\
\hline
160 \\
154 \\
\hline
60 \\
44 \\
\hline
16
\end{array}
$$

- Move the decimal point two places to the right, and round to the nearest tenth:

$$0.2272 = 22.7\%$$

Finding a number when you know a percentage of it

- An example of finding a number when you know a percentage of it is "70% of what number is 7?" To solve, follow these steps:

  – First, convert 70% into a decimal fraction by removing the percent sign and moving the decimal point two places to the left:

$$70\% = 0.70$$

  – Next, divide 7 by 0.70. Move the decimal two places to the right in both the divisor (to make it a whole number) and the dividend. The quotient is 10:

$$
\begin{array}{r}
10.0 \\
0.70\overline{)7.00\,0}
\end{array}
$$

Learn by example

The patient received 600 ml of I.V. fluid out of 1,000 ml that was ordered. What percentage of I.V. fluid did the patient receive?

- What you really want to find out is "600 is what percentage of 1,000?"
- First, restate it as a division problem, with 600 as the dividend and 1,000 as the divisor:

$$
\begin{array}{r}
0.60 \\
1000\overline{)600.00} \\
\underline{600\ 0} \\
00
\end{array}
$$

- Next, move the decimal point in the quotient two places to the right and add a percentage sign:

$$0.60 = 60\%$$

So, 600 is 60% of 1,000.

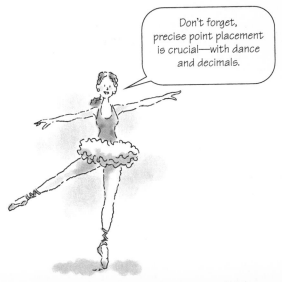

Don't forget, precise point placement is crucial—with dance and decimals.

Using ratios and proportions

- A ratio is a numeric way of comparing two items.
  - For example, if 100 syringes come in 1 box, then the number of syringes compared to the number of boxes is 100 to 1.
  - A ratio is written with a colon to separate the numbers (such as 100:1).
  - The same comparison can be made using a fraction ($\frac{100}{1}$).
- A proportion is a statement of equality between two ratios.
  - It can be expressed with either ratios (using double colons to separate the ratios) or fractions.

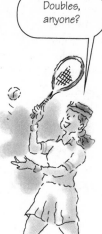

Doubles, anyone?

Learn by example

If the ratio of syringes to boxes is 100:1, then 200 syringes are provided in 2 boxes.

- Use double colons to represent equality between the ratios:

      100 syringes : 1 box :: 200 syringes : 2 boxes

  or

      100 : 1 :: 200 : 2

- Using fractions, this same comparison can be written as follows:

$$\frac{100 \text{ syringes}}{1 \text{ box}} = \frac{200 \text{ syringes}}{2 \text{ boxes}}$$

  or

$$\frac{100}{1} = \frac{200}{2}$$

Solving for *X*

- Sometimes, part of a ratio or fraction is unknown or incomplete.
- In this case, an equation can be set up using an *X* to represent the unknown part.

X marks what spot?

Being able to find the value of *X* is vital in making dosage calculations. For example, suppose a practitioner orders a drug for your patient but the drug isn't available in the ordered strength. How do you decide on the right amount of drug to administer?

Here's how

Suppose you receive an order to administer 0.1 mg of epinephrine subcutaneously, but the only epinephrine on hand is a 1-ml ampule that contains 1 mg of epinephrine. To calculate the volume for injection, state the problem in a proportion:

$$1 \text{ mg} : 1 \text{ ml} :: 0.1 \text{ mg} : X \text{ ml}$$

Rewrite the problem as an equation by applying the principle that the product of the means (numbers in the middle of the proportion) equals the product of the extremes (numbers at either end of the proportion).

$$1 \text{ ml} \times 0.1 \text{ mg} = 1 \text{ mg} \times X \text{ ml}$$

Solve for *X* by dividing both sides of the equation by the known value that appears on the same side of the equation as the unknown value *X*. Then cancel out units that appear in the numerator and denominator. (This isolates *X* on one side of the equation.)

$$\frac{1 \text{ ml} \times 0.1 \text{ \sout{mg}}}{1 \text{ \sout{mg}}} = \frac{1 \text{ \sout{mg}} \times X \text{ ml}}{1 \text{ \sout{mg}}}$$

$$X = 0.1 \text{ ml}$$

Solving common-fraction equations

In addition to X, there are many things you could call "unknown."

- Common-fraction equations form the basis for solving other simple equations to find the value of X.

Learn by example

Solve for X.

$$X = \frac{1}{5} \times \frac{3}{9}$$

- Multiply the numerators:

$$1 \times 3 = 3$$

- Multiply the denominators:

$$5 \times 9 = 45$$

- Restate the equation with the new information:

$$X = \frac{1 \times 3}{5 \times 9} = \frac{3}{45}$$

- Reduce the fraction by dividing the numerator and denominator by the lowest common denominator (3):

$$X = \frac{3 \div 3}{45 \div 3} = \frac{1}{15}$$

- Convert the fraction to a decimal fraction by dividing the numerator by the denominator. Round off to the nearest hundredth:

$$X = \frac{1}{15} = 1 \div 15 = 0.07$$

Calculation clues

Making whole numbers fractions

You can change any whole number into a fraction by making the whole number the numerator and placing it over a 1, which is the denominator. The value of the number doesn't change.

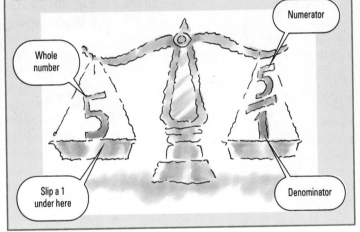

Learn by example

Solve for X when the whole number is 3.

$$X = \frac{125}{500} \times 3$$

- Convert the whole number 3 into the fraction $^3/_1$:

$$X = \frac{125}{500} \times \frac{3}{1}$$

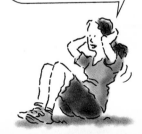

If only reducing my waistline was as simple as reducing fractions!

- Reduce $^{125}/_{500}$ by dividing the numerator and denominator by the lowest common denominator (125). The equation becomes:

$$X = \frac{125 \div 125}{500 \div 125} \times \frac{3}{1}$$

or

$$X = \frac{1}{4} \times \frac{3}{1}$$

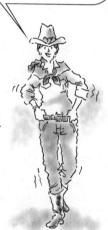

I know this problem seems mighty long, but once you get the hang of it, you'll be two-steppin' through equations with the best of 'em.

- Multiply the numerators:

$$1 \times 3 = 3$$

- Multiply the denominators:

$$4 \times 1 = 4$$

- Restate the equation with this new information:

$$X = \frac{1 \times 3}{4 \times 1} \times \frac{3}{4}$$

- The fraction $\frac{3}{4}$ can't be reduced further. Convert it into a decimal fraction:

$$X = \frac{3}{4} = 3 \div 4 = 0.75$$

Solving decimal-fraction equations

- This method for solving decimal-fraction equations is similar to that used for common-fraction equations.
- Just remember to move the decimal point to convert to a fraction.

Learn by example

Solve for X.

$$X = \frac{0.05}{0.02} \times 3$$

- First, eliminate the decimal points by moving them two spaces to the right. Then remove the zeros:

$$X = {}^{5}\!/_{2} \times 3$$

- Next, convert the whole number 3 into a fraction:

$$X = \frac{5}{2} \times \frac{3}{1}$$

- Now multiply the numerators:

$$5 \times 3 = 15$$

- Multiply the denominators:

$$2 \times 1 = 2$$

- Restate the equation with this new information:

$$X = \frac{5 \times 3}{2 \times 1} \times \frac{15}{2}$$

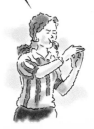

Time out for decimal conversions!

- The fraction ${}^{15}\!/_{2}$ can't be reduced further. Convert it into a decimal fraction:

$$X = \frac{15}{2} = 15 \div 2 = 7.5$$

Learn by example

Solve for X in this equation.

$$X = \frac{0.33}{0.11} \times 0.6$$

- Remove the decimal point by moving it two spaces to the right. Then remove the zeros:

$$X = \frac{33}{11} \times 0.6$$

- Convert 0.6 into a fraction:

$$X = \frac{33}{11} \times \frac{0.6}{1}$$

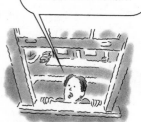

Hang in there! You'll have this problem solved in no time. Me, on the other hand...

- Multiply the numerators:

$$33 \times 0.6 = 19.8$$

- Multiply the denominators:

$$11 \times 1 = 11$$

- Restate the equation with this new information:

$$X = \frac{33 \times 0.6}{11 \times 1} = \frac{19.8}{11}$$

- The fraction $^{19.8}/11$ can't be reduced further. Convert it into a decimal fraction:

$$X = \frac{19.8}{11} = 19.8 \div 11 = 1.8$$

Solving proportion problems with ratios

- A proportion can be written with ratios, as in:

$$4{:}1 :: 20{:}5$$

- The outer numbers are called the *extremes*.

- The inner numbers are called the *means*.
- The product of the means equals the product of the extremes:

$$1 \times 20 = 4 \times 5$$

Learn by example

Solve for X in this example.

$$4{:}8 :: 8{:}X$$

- Rewrite the problem so that the means and extremes are multiplied:

$$8 \times 8 = 4 \times X$$

- Obtain the products of the means and extremes, and put them into an equation:

$$64 = 4X$$

- Solve for X by dividing both sides by 4. This will isolate X on one side of the equation:

$$\frac{64}{4} = \frac{4X}{4}$$

- Find X:

$$64 \div 4 = X$$

or

$$X = 16$$

- Replace X with 16, and restate the proportion in ratios:

$$4{:}8 :: 8{:}16$$

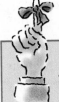

Memory jogger

When working with ratios, the product of the means always equals the product of the extremes. To differentiate these terms, remember:

means are middle numbers

extremes are end numbers.

That's extreme, dude!

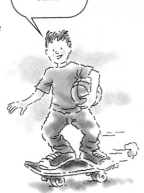

Learn by example

Solve for X in this proportion.

$$X{:}12 :: 6{:}24$$

- Rewrite the problem so that the means and extremes are multiplied:

$$12 \times 6 = X \times 24$$

- Obtain the products of the means and extremes, and put them into an equation:

$$72 = 24X$$

- Solve for X by dividing both sides by 24 (this isolates X on one side of the equation):

$$\frac{72}{24} = \frac{24X}{24}$$

- Find X:

$$72 \div 24 = X$$

$$\text{or}$$

$$X = 3$$

- Now replace X with 3, and restate the proportion in ratios:

$$3{:}12 :: 6{:}24$$

Get down with da means and extremes!

Solving proportion problems with fractions

- In a proportion expressed as a fraction, cross products are equal.
- The position of X doesn't matter.

Calculation clues

Cross product principle

In a proportion expressed as fractions, cross products are equal. In other words, the numerator on the equation's left side multiplied by the denominator on the equation's right side equals the denominator on the equation's left side multiplied by the numerator on the equation's right side.

This statement has a lot of words. The same meaning is communicated more simply in the illustration below left.

Applies to ratios as well

Note that the same principle applies to ratios. In a proportion expressed as ratios, the product of the **m**eans (numbers in the **m**iddle) equals the product of the **e**xtremes (numbers on the **e**nds). Consider the illustration below right.

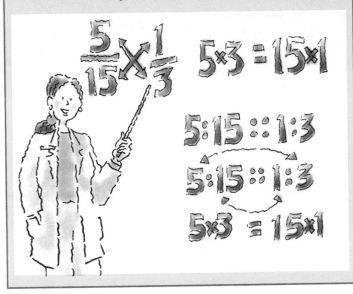

Calculation clues

Cross products to the rescue

Fractions can be used to describe the relative proportion of ingredients—for example, the amount of a drug relative to its solution.

Suppose you have a vial containing 10 mg/ml of morphine. You can write this fraction to describe it:

> **Amount of drug** — 10 mg

$$\frac{10 \text{ mg}}{1 \text{ ml}}$$

> **Amount of solution** — 1 ml

The plot thickens

Now suppose you need to administer 8 mg of morphine to your patient. How much of the solution should you use?

1. Write a second fraction, using X to represent the amount of solution:

> **An unknown quantity** — X ml

$$\frac{8 \text{ mg}}{X \text{ ml}}$$

2. Set up the equation. Keep the fractions in the same relative proportion of drug to solution.

3. Rewrite the problem so that cross products are multiplied:

> **Cross-multiply**

$$\frac{10 \text{ mg}}{1 \text{ ml}} \bowtie \frac{8 \text{ mg}}{X \text{ ml}}$$

4. This gives you:

$$10X = 8$$

5. Solve for X by dividing both sides by 10, and you're left with:

$$X = \frac{8}{10}$$

6. Convert this to a decimal fraction because you'll be drawing up medication and need to work with a decimal:

$$X = 0.8 \text{ ml}$$

> **The answer**

This is how much of the morphine you should use.

Learn by example

Practice solving for X in this equation.

$$\frac{3}{4} = \frac{9}{X}$$

- Rewrite the problem so the cross products are multiplied:

$$3 \times X = 4 \times 9$$

- Obtain the cross products and put them into an equation:

$$3X = 36$$

- Solve for X by dividing both sides by 3. This isolates X on one side of the equation:

$$\frac{3X}{3} = \frac{36}{3}$$

- Find X:

$$X = \frac{36}{3}$$

$$\text{or, } X = 12$$

- Replace X with 12, and restate the proportions in fractions:

$$\frac{3}{4} = \frac{9}{12}$$

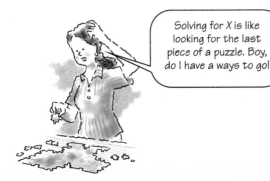

Solving for X is like looking for the last piece of a puzzle. Boy, do I have a ways to go!

Dimensional analysis

- Also called *factor analysis* or *factor labeling*, dimensional analysis is a six-step method of solving equations.
- It involves arranging a series of ratios (called *factors*) into a fractional equation.
- Each factor contains two quantities of measurement that are related to each other.
- Some problems contain all the information needed to identify the factors, set up the equation, and find the solution; some require a conversion factor.

Six-step method
Learn by example

Use these six steps to determine how many feet are in 48 inches.

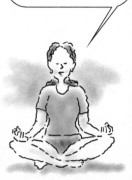

> I wonder if this is a form of transcendental dimensional analysis?

✌️ *Given quantity*—Identify the quantity given in the problem (48 inches).

✌️ *Wanted quantity*—Identify the quantity wanted in the problem as an unknown unit; this will be the answer (*X* feet).

✌️ *Conversion factor*—Find the equivalents necessary to convert between systems (12 inches = 1 foot).

✌️ *Problem*—Set up the problem using necessary equivalents. Make sure that the units you want to cancel out are in both a numerator and a denominator:

$$\frac{48 \text{ inches}}{1} \times \frac{1 \text{ foot}}{12 \text{ inches}}$$

Help desk

Following the steps

Remember these steps when calculating an equation using dimensional analysis, and you'll soon be standing on top of a solution.

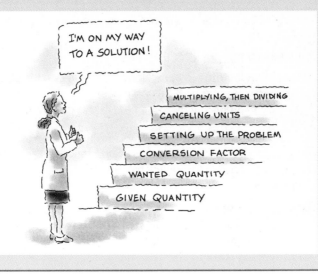

Cancellation—Cancel units that appear in the numerator and denominator to isolate the unit you're seeking:

$$\frac{48 \ \cancel{\text{inches}}}{1} \times \frac{1 \ \text{foot}}{12 \ \cancel{\text{inches}}}$$

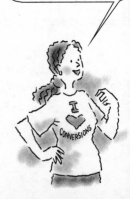

Multiplying and dividing—Multiply the numerators and then the denominators; then divide the product of the numerators by the product of the denominators to reach the wanted quantity:

$$\frac{48}{1} \times \frac{1 \text{ foot}}{12} = \frac{48 \times 1 \text{ foot}}{1 \times 12} = \frac{48 \text{ feet}}{12} = 4 \text{ feet}$$

There are 4 feet in 48 inches.

Conversion factors

- Conversion factors are equivalents between two measurement systems or units of measurement.
- Common examples include 1 day = 24 hours and 12 inches = 1 foot.
- Because quantities and unit of measurement are equivalent, they can serve as the numerator or denominator. For example, the conversion for inches to feet can be written as $^{12}/_1$ or $^1/_{12}$.

Learn by example

If a package weighs 38 ounces (oz), what is its weight in pounds (lb)?

- Identify the quantity:

  38 oz

- Identify the wanted quantity:

  X lb

- Find the conversion factor:

  1 lb = 16 oz

- Set up the problem:

$$\frac{38 \text{ oz}}{1} \times \frac{1 \text{ lb}}{16 \text{ oz}}$$

You need not have an aversion to conversions. They can be incredibly easy!

- Cancel units that appear in both the numerator and denominator:

$$\frac{38 \ \cancel{oz}}{1} \times \frac{1 \ lb}{16 \ \cancel{oz}}$$

- Multiply the numerators and denominators; then divide the products:

$$\frac{38 \times 1 \ lb}{1 \times 16} = \frac{38 \ lb}{16} = 2.4 \ lb$$

The package weighs 2.4 lb.

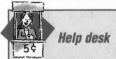

Help desk

Common conversion factors

Keep this chart handy for quick reference to breeze through problems that call for these common conversions.

1 kg	=	2.2 lb
16 oz	=	1 lb
8 oz	=	1 cup
1 oz	=	30 ml
1 tsp	=	5 ml
1 grain	=	60 mg
12 inches	=	1 foot
3 feet	=	1 yd

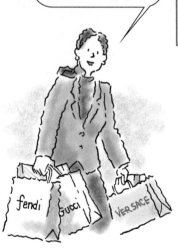

I don't even want to guess what these packages weigh...

fendi   Gucci   VERSACE

Learn by example

How much would the same package weigh in kilograms (kg)?

• Identify the given:

$$38 \text{ oz}$$

• Identify the wanted:

$$X \text{ kg}$$

• Identify the conversion factor—there are two in this case:

$$1 \text{ lb} = 16 \text{ oz}$$

$$1 \text{ kg} = 2.2 \text{ lb}$$

• Set up the problem:

$$\frac{38 \text{ oz}}{1} \times \frac{1 \text{ lb}}{16 \text{ oz}} = \frac{1 \text{ kg}}{2.2 \text{ lb}}$$

• Cancel units that appear in both the numerator and denominator:

$$\frac{38 \text{ \cancel{oz}}}{1} \times \frac{1 \text{ \cancel{lb}}}{16 \text{ \cancel{oz}}} = \frac{1 \text{ kg}}{2.2 \text{ \cancel{lb}}}$$

• Multiply the numerators and denominators, then divide the products:

$$\frac{38 \times 1 \times 1}{1 \times 16 \times 2.2} = \frac{38 \text{ kg}}{35.2} = 1.08 \text{ kg}$$

The package weighs 1.08 kg.

Learn by example

The practitioner prescribes 10,000 units of heparin added to 500 ml of D_5W at 1,200 units/hour. How many drops (gtt) per minute should you administer if the I.V. tubing delivers 10 gtt/minute?

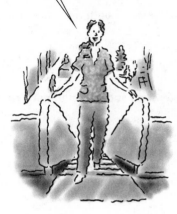

- Determine the given quantities (there are three in this case):

    ☝ 1st quantity: $\dfrac{10 \text{ gtt}}{1 \text{ ml}}$

    ✌ 2nd quantity: $\dfrac{500 \text{ ml}}{10,000 \text{ units}}$

    🖖 3rd quantity: $\dfrac{1,200 \text{ units}}{1 \text{ hr}}$

- Determine the wanted quantity:

    X gtt/minute

- Use the conversion factor:

    $1 \text{ hour} = 60 \text{ minutes}$ or $\dfrac{1 \text{ hr}}{60 \text{ minutes}}$

- Set up the problem:

$$\frac{10 \text{ gtt}}{1 \text{ ml}} \times \frac{500 \text{ ml}}{10,000 \text{ units}} \times \frac{1,200 \text{ units}}{1 \text{ hr}} \times \frac{1 \text{ hr}}{60 \text{ minutes}}$$

- Cancel units that appear in both the numerator and denominator:

$$\frac{10 \text{ gtt}}{1 \text{ \cancel{ml}}} \times \frac{500 \text{ \cancel{ml}}}{10,000 \text{ \cancel{units}}} \times \frac{1,200 \text{ \cancel{units}}}{1 \text{ \cancel{hr}}} \times \frac{1 \text{ \cancel{hr}}}{60 \text{ minutes}}$$

- Multiply the numerators and denominators; then divide the products:

$$\frac{10 \times 500 \times 1,200 \text{ gtt}}{10,000 \times 60 \text{ minutes}} = \frac{6,000,000 \text{ gtt}}{600,000 \text{ minutes}} = 10 \text{ gtt/minute}$$

The heparin should be administered at 10 gtt/minute.

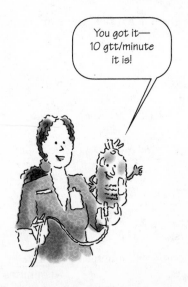

You got it—
10 gtt/minute
it is!

Measurement systems

2

Metric system

- A decimal system of measurement (based on the number 10 and multiples and subdivisions of 10); the most widely used system for measuring drugs
- Has three basic units of measurement

☞ *Meter* (m) is the basic unit of length.

What a little prefix can do

In the metric system, the addition of a prefix to one of the basic units of measure indicates a multiple or subdivision of that unit. Here's a list of prefixes, abbreviations, and multiples and subdivisions of each unit.

Prefix	Abbreviation	Multiples and subdivisions
kilo	k	1,000
hecto	h	100
deka	dk	10
deci	d	0.1 ($\frac{1}{10}$)
centi	c	0.01 ($\frac{1}{100}$)
milli	m	0.001 ($\frac{1}{1,000}$)
micro	mc	0.000001 ($\frac{1}{1,000,000}$)
nano	n	0.000000001 ($\frac{1}{1,000,000,000}$)
pico	p	0.000000000001 ($\frac{1}{1,000,000,000,000}$)

Liter (L) is the basic unit of volume.

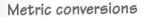 *Gram* (g) is the basic unit of weight.

- Uses prefixes to designate multiples and subdivisions (or fractions) of basic units

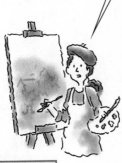

Did you know that the metric system was developed in France in the 1700s?

Metric conversions

- To convert from a smaller unit to a larger unit (multiple), move the decimal point to the left.
- To convert from a larger unit to a smaller unit (subdivision), move the decimal point to the right.

Insta-metric conversion table

Want a quick and easy way to jump back and forth between different metric measures? Just use the fantastic "insta-metric" table below. Make a copy of it to post in a conspicuous spot on your unit. Always remember, a milliliter is to a liter as a microgram is to a milligram.

Liquids	Solids
1 ml = 1 cm^3 (or cc)	1,000 mcg = 1 mg
1,000 ml = 1 L	1,000 mg = 1 g
100 cl = 1 L	100 cg = 1 g
10 dl = 1 L	10 dg = 1 g
10 L = 1 dkl	10 g = 1 dkg
100 L = 1 hl	100 g = 1 hg
1,000 L = 1 kl	1,000 g = 1 kg

Amazing metric decimal place finder

When performing metric conversions, use this scale as a guide to decimal placement. Each bar represents one decimal place.

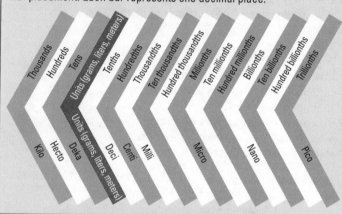

Learn by example: Using the *Amazing metric decimal place finder*

Convert 15 meters (m) to kilometers (km).

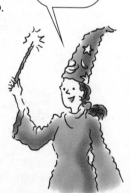

Amazing, isn't it?!

- Count the number of places to the right or left of *meters* it takes to reach *kilo*. (*Kilo* is three places to the left, indicating that a kilometer is 1,000 times larger than a meter.)
- Move the decimal place in the number 15 (15.0) three places to the left, and you get 0.015 km. So, 15 m = 0.015 km. (Remember to place a zero in front of the decimal point to draw attention to the decimal point's presence.)

Learn by example: Using the prefix chart

Convert 15 meters (m) to kilometers (km).

- Find the multiple corresponding with *kilo* on the chart (in this case, the multiple is 1,000).
- To go from a smaller unit to a larger unit, divide by the multiple; so divide 15 m by 1,000 (this can be set up as an equation):

$$X = \frac{15 \text{ m}}{1,000}$$

$$X = 0.015 \text{ km}$$

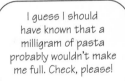

...and three to the left and twirl!

Learn by example: Using the *Amazing metric decimal place finder*

Convert 5 g to milligrams.

- Count the number of places from *grams* to *milli* on the chart. (*Milli* is three places to the right, indicating that a milligram is 1,000 times smaller than a gram.)
- Move the decimal point in 5 (5.0) three places to the right, and you get 5,000. So, 5 g = 5,000 mg.

I guess I should have known that a milligram of pasta probably wouldn't make me full. Check, please!

Learn by example: Using the prefix chart

Convert 5 g to milligrams.

- Find the subdivision corresponding with *milli* on the chart (in this case, it's 0.001, or ¹⁄₁,₀₀₀).
- Set up an equation to convert grams to milligrams by dividing

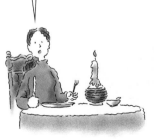

5 g by $\frac{1}{1,000}$ (remember, when dividing fractions, you need to invert the divisor and multiply by this reciprocal):

$$\frac{5 \text{ g}}{\frac{1}{1,000}}$$

$$X = 5 \text{ g} \times 1,000$$

$$X = 5,000 \text{ mg}$$

$$5 \text{ g} = 5,000 \text{ mg}$$

Solving for X

• Another way to convert between metric units is to solve for X (alternatively, you can use the ratio-and-proportion method).

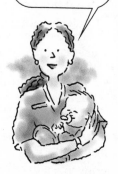

Never before was holding 6.5 kg such a joy!

• Follow the same principles of substituting X for the unknown quantity as discussed in chapter 1.
• Remember: to add, subtract, multiply, or divide different metric units, first convert all quantities to the same units.

Learn by example

An infant weighs 6.5 kg. How much does he weigh in grams?

• Referring to the *Insta-metric conversion table*, you'll see that 1,000 g equals 1 kg.
• Set up the equation, substituting X for the unknown weight in grams:

$$\frac{1,000 \text{ g}}{1 \text{ kg}} = \frac{X}{6.5 \text{ kg}}$$

- Cross-multiply the fractions:

$$\frac{1,000 \text{ g}}{1 \text{ kg}} \bowtie \frac{X}{6.5 \text{ kg}}$$

$$X \times 1 \text{ kg} = 6.5 \text{ kg} \times 1,000 \text{ g}$$

- Divide both sides of the equation by 1 kg to isolate X:

$$\frac{X \times 1 \text{ \cancel{kg}}}{1 \text{ \cancel{kg}}} = \frac{6.5 \text{ \cancel{kg}} \times 1,000 \text{ g}}{1 \text{ \cancel{kg}}}$$

$$X = 6,500 \text{ g}$$

The infant weighs 6,500 g.

Calculation clues

Overcoming fear of fractions

If you don't like working with fractions, here's an alternative to solving for X in problems. In the example about determining an infant's weight in grams (above), the equation that's expressed in fractions can also be set up as a ratio and proportion:

$$1,000 \text{ g} : 1 \text{ kg} :: X : 6.5 \text{ kg}$$

- Multiply the means and extremes:

$$X \times 1 \text{ kg} = 1,000 \text{ g} \times 6.5 \text{ kg}$$

- Divide both sides of the equation by 1 kg to isolate X.
- Cancel units that appear in both the numerator and denominator.

$$X = 6,500 \text{ g}$$

The infant weighs 6,500 g.

Learn by example

If a patient received 0.375 L of lactated Ringer's solution, how many milliliters did he receive?

- Referring to the *Insta-metric conversion table*, note that 1 L equals 1,000 ml.
- Set up the equation, substituting X for the unknown amount of I.V. solution in milliliters:

$$\frac{1\,L}{1,000\,ml} = \frac{0.375\,L}{X}$$

- Cross-multiply the fractions:

$$\frac{1\,L}{1,000\,ml} \bowtie \frac{0.375\,L}{X}$$

$$X \times 1\,L = 0.375\,L \times 1,000\,ml$$

- Divide both sides of the equation by 1 L to isolate X:

$$\frac{X \times \cancel{1\,L}}{\cancel{1\,L}} = \frac{0.375\,L \times 1,000\,ml}{1\,\cancel{L}}$$

$$X = 375\,ml$$

The patient received 375 ml of I.V. fluid.

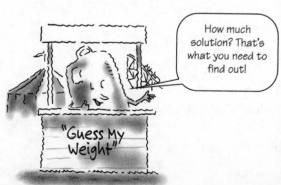

How much solution? That's what you need to find out!

"Guess My Weight"

Learn by example

Add 2 kg, 202 mg, and 222 g, expressing the total in grams.

- First, convert all the measurements to grams:
  - 1 kg = 1,000 g; therefore, multiply 2 kg by 1,000 to get 2,000 g.
  - 1,000 mg = 1 g, and 1 mg = $\frac{1}{1,000}$ g; therefore, divide 202 mg by 1,000 to get 0.202 g.
- Now do the addition:

$$2,000 + 0.202 + 222 = 2,222.202 \text{ g}$$

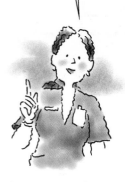

Remember to convert to like units before completing the problem.

Apothecaries' system

- Used before adoption of the metric system (rarely used today)
- Only used to measure liquid volume and solid weight
  - Basic unit for measuring liquid volume is the dram (fluidram).
  - Basic unit for measuring solid weight is the grain.
- Includes some common household measurements (ounce, pint, quart, gallon)
- Traditionally uses Roman numerals

Roman numeral conversions

- In pharmacologic application, Roman numerals ss (½) through X (10) are written in lower case.
- Unit of measurement goes before the numeral; for example, 5 grains is written as *grains v.*

Ye olde apothecaries' system

The apothecaries' system uses these units to measure liquid volume and solid weight.

Liquid volume	Solid weight
60 minims (m) = 1 fluidram	60 grains (gr) = 1 dram
8 fluidrams = 1 fluid ounce (oz)	8 drams = 1 oz
16 fluid oz = 1 pint (pt)	12 oz = 1 pound (lb)
2 pt = 1 quart (qt)	
4 qt = 1 gallon (gal)	

- When a smaller numeral precedes a larger numeral, subtract the smaller numeral from the larger numeral:

$$IX = 10 - 1 = 9$$

- When a smaller numeral follows a larger numeral, add the numerals:

$$XI = 10 + 1 = 11$$

- To convert an Arabic numeral to a Roman numeral, break the Arabic numeral into its parts and then translate each part into Roman numerals:

$$36 = 30 + 6 = XXX + VI = XXXVI$$

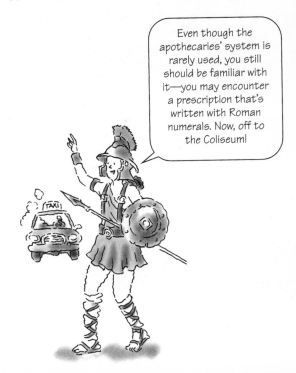

Even though the apothecaries' system is rarely used, you still should be familiar with it—you may encounter a prescription that's written with Roman numerals. Now, off to the Coliseum!

The road to Roman numerals

Here's a handy review of Roman numerals.

½ = ss	11 = XI	30 = XXX
1 = I	12 = XII	40 = XL
2 = II	13 = XIII	50 = L
3 = III	14 = XIV	60 = LX
4 = IV	15 = XV	70 = LXX
5 = V	16 = XVI	80 = LXXX
6 = VI	17 = XVII	90 = XC
7 = VII	18 = XVIII	100 = C
8 = VIII	19 = XIX	500 = D
9 = IX	20 = XX	1,000 = M
10 = X		

Household system

- Uses droppers, teaspoons, tablespoons, and cups to measure liquid medication doses
- Useful only for approximate measurements because devices aren't all alike (for exact measurements, use the metric system)

A spoonful of sugar

Mary Poppins was no pharmacist, but she knew how to make the medicine go down. She recommended a spoonful of sugar. The question is, how much is in a spoonful?

Here's a rundown of the most commonly used household units of measure and their equivalent liquid volumes. *Note:* Don't use the abbreviations "t" for teaspoon and "T" for tablespoon because it's easy to make errors when writing them quickly.

60 drops (gtt)	=	1 teaspoon (tsp)
3 tsp	=	1 tablespoon (tbs)
2 tbs	=	1 ounce (oz)
8 oz	=	1 cup
16 oz (2 cups)	=	1 pint (pt)
2 pt	=	1 quart (qt)
4 qt	=	1 gallon (gal)

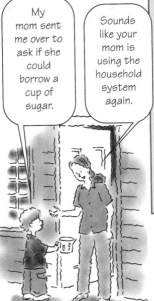

My mom sent me over to ask if she could borrow a cup of sugar.

Sounds like your mom is using the household system again.

Making sure the cup doesn't runneth over

Will your patient be taking medication at home? If so, teach him to use the devices below to help ensure accurate measurements.

Medication cup

A medication cup is calibrated in household, metric, and apothecaries' systems. Tell the patient to set the cup on a counter or flat surface and to check the fluid measurement at eye level.

Dropper

A dropper is calibrated in household or metric systems or in terms of medication strength or concentration. Advise the patient to hold the dropper at eye level to check the fluid measurement.

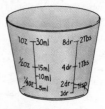

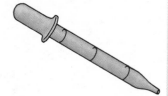

Hollow-handle spoon

A hollow-handle spoon is calibrated in teaspoons and tablespoons. Teach the patient to check the dose after filling by holding the spoon upright at eye level. Instruct him to administer the medication by tilting the spoon until the medicine fills the bowl of the spoon and then placing the spoon in his mouth.

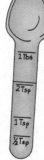

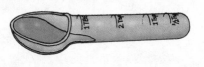

Household system conversions

- To convert within the household system, follow the same principles of solving for X as described previously.
- Conversion to another system (such as household or metric) is also possible.

Learn by example

The practitioner has ordered 120 drops (gtt) of an expectorant cough syrup every 6 hours for your patient. The drug label gives instructions in teaspoons. How many teaspoons should you administer?

- There are 60 gtt of liquid in 1 teaspoon (tsp). Set up an equation as follows to find out how many teaspoons are in 120 gtt, using X as the unknown quantity:

$$\frac{60 \text{ gtt}}{1 \text{ tsp}} = \frac{120 \text{ gtt}}{X}$$

- Cross-multiply the fractions:

$$X \times 60 \text{ gtt} = 1 \text{ tsp} \times 120 \text{ gtt}$$

- Solve for X by dividing both sides of the equation by 60 gtt:

$$\frac{X \times \cancel{60 \text{ gtt}}}{\cancel{60 \text{ gtt}}} = \frac{1 \text{ tsp} \times 120 \cancel{\text{ gtt}}}{60 \cancel{\text{ gtt}}}$$

$$X = \frac{1 \text{ tsp} \times 120}{60}$$

$$X = 2 \text{ tsp}$$

The patient should receive 2 tsp of cough syrup.

Avoirdupois system

- Means *goods sold by weight*
- Used for ordering and purchasing some pharmaceutical products and for measuring patients
- Units of measurement: grains (gr), ounces (oz), and pounds (lb)
  - 1 oz = 480 gr
  - 1 lb = 16 oz (or 7,680 gr)
- Measurement of pound (16 oz) different from that used in apothecaries' system (12 oz)

Avoirdupois system conversions

- To convert within the avoirdupois system, simply solve for X.
- Conversion to apothecaries' or metric system is also possible.

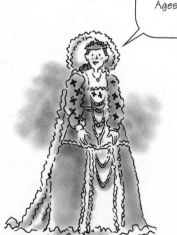

The avoirdupois system has been around since about the Middle Ages...a very, very long time, indeed!

Measure for measure

Here are some approximate liquid and solid equivalents among the household, apothecaries', avoirdupois, and metric systems. Use your facility's protocol for converting measurements from one system to another.

Liquids

Household	Apothecaries'	Metric
1 drop (gtt)	1 minim (m)	0.06 milliliter (ml)
15 to 16 gtt	15 to 16 m	1 ml
1 teaspoon (tsp)	1 fluidram	5 ml
1 tablespoon (tbs)	½ fluid ounce (oz)	15 ml
2 tbs	1 fluid oz	30 ml
1 cup	8 fluid oz	240 ml
1 pint (pt)	16 fluid oz	480 ml
1 quart (qt)	32 fluid oz	960 ml
1 gallon (gal)	128 fluid oz	3,840 ml

Solids

Avoirdupois	Apothecaries'	Metric
1 grain (gr)	1 gr	0.06 gram (g)
1 gr	1 gr	60 milligrams (mg)
15.4 gr	15 gr	1 g
1 oz	480 grains	28.35 g
1 pound (lb)	1.33 lb	454 g
2.2 lb	2.7 lb	1 kilogram (kg)

Learn by example

How many pounds are in 32 ounces?

- There are 16 ounces in 1 pound. To find out how many pounds are in 32 ounces, set up the following equation using X as the unknown quantity:

$$\frac{16 \text{ oz}}{1 \text{ lb}} = \frac{32 \text{ oz}}{X}$$

- Cross-multiply the fractions:

$$X \times 16 \text{ oz} = 32 \text{ oz} \times 1 \text{ lb}$$

- Solve for X by dividing both sides of the equation by 16 oz:

$$\frac{X \times \cancel{16 \text{ oz}}}{\cancel{16 \text{ oz}}} = \frac{32 \cancel{\text{ oz}} \times 1 \text{ lb}}{16 \cancel{\text{ oz}}}$$

$$X = 1 \text{ lb} \times 2$$

$$X = 2 \text{ lb}$$

There are 2 lb in 32 oz.

Unit system

- Only used for certain drugs
  - Insulin (most common), heparin, bacitracin, and penicillins G and V
  - Some hormones and vitamins
- Unique unit of measurement for each drug

Unit system conversions

- To calculate the dose to be administered when a medication is available in units, use this equation:

$$\frac{\text{amount of drug in ml or other measure}}{\text{dose required in units}} = \frac{\text{1 ml or other measure}}{\text{drug available in units}}$$

Remember that units are unique to individual drugs. So make sure you know what type of unit goes with each drug you administer.

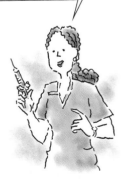

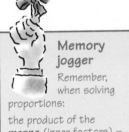

Memory jogger

Remember, when solving proportions:

the product of the **means** (inner factors) = the product of the **extremes** (outer factors).

Learn by example

A standard heparin drip of 25,000 units in 500 ml of half-normal saline solution is ordered for your patient. The heparin vial that's available has 5,000 units/ml. How many milliliters of heparin should you add to the I.V. fluid?

• Set up a proportion using X as the unknown quantity:

$$\frac{X}{25,000 \text{ units}} = \frac{1 \text{ ml}}{5,000 \text{ units}}$$

• Cross-multiply the fractions:

$$X \times 5,000 \text{ units} = 1 \text{ ml} \times 25,000 \text{ units}$$

• Find X by dividing both sides of the equation by 5,000 units:

$$\frac{X \times \cancel{5,000 \text{ units}}}{\cancel{5,000 \text{ units}}} = \frac{1 \text{ ml} \times 25,000 \cancel{\text{ units}}}{5,000 \cancel{\text{ units}}}$$

$$X = 5 \text{ ml}$$

You should add 5 ml of heparin to the I.V. fluid.

Milliequivalent system

- Used with some electrolytes, such as potassium and sodium
- Information about the number of milliequivalents (mEq) in a milliliter provided by individual drug manufacturers

Milliequivalent system conversions

- To calculate the dose to be given when a medication is available in milliequivalents, use this equation:

$$\frac{\text{amount of drug in ml or other measure}}{\text{dose required in mEq}} = \frac{\text{1 ml or other measure}}{\text{drug available in mEq}}$$

Learn by example

Your patient needs 25 mEq of sodium bicarbonate. The vial from the pharmacy contains 50 mEq in 50 ml. How many milliliters of the solution should you administer?

- Set up a proportion using X as the unknown quantity:

$$\frac{X}{25 \text{ mEq}} = \frac{50 \text{ ml}}{50 \text{ mEq}}$$

- Cross-multiply the fractions:

$$X \times 50 \text{ mEq} = 50 \text{ ml} \times 25 \text{ mEq}$$

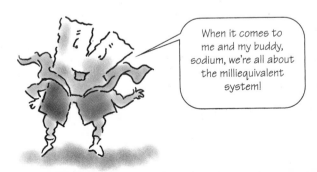

When it comes to me and my buddy, sodium, we're all about the milliequivalent system!

• Find X by dividing both sides of the equation by 50 mEq:

$$\frac{X \times \cancel{50\ mEq}}{\cancel{50\ mEq}} = \frac{50\ ml \times 25\ \cancel{mEq}}{50\ \cancel{mEq}}$$

$$X = 25\ ml$$

You should administer 25 ml of sodium bicarbonate solution.

Frequently used conversions

- To convert from one system to another, know the equivalent measures.
- The most commonly used conversions are for kilograms to pounds and inches to centimeters:
  - 1 kg = 2.2 lb
  - 1″ = 2.54 cm

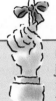

Memory jogger

Remember this jingle when converting inches to centimeters and vice versa:

"2.54, that's 1 inch and no more!"

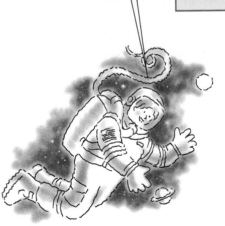

Outer space…the final frontier! Any guesses on how much I weigh out here?

Learn by example

To prepare medications for your hypotensive patient, you must determine her weight in kilograms. You know that she weighs 125 lb, but how much is this in kilograms?

- Set up a proportion using X as the unknown weight:

$$\frac{X}{125\ lb} = \frac{1\ kg}{2.2\ lb}$$

- Cross-multiply the fractions:

$$X \times 2.2\ lb = 1\ kg \times 125\ lb$$

- Find X by dividing both sides of the equation by 2.2 lb:

$$\frac{X \times \cancel{2.2\ lb}}{\cancel{2.2\ lb}} = \frac{1\ kg \times 125\ \cancel{lb}}{2.2\ \cancel{lb}}$$

$$X = 56.8\ kg$$

Your patient weighs 56.8 kg.

I prefer to express my weight in kilograms.

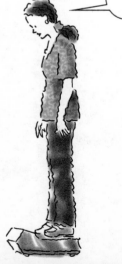

Recording drug administration

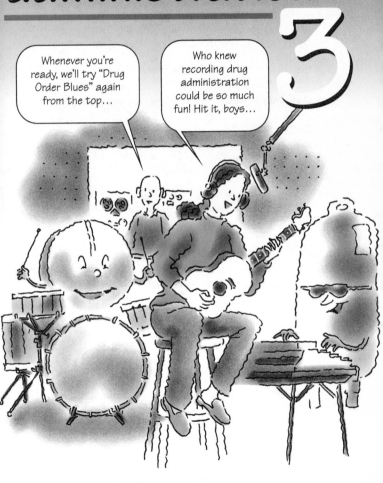

Drug orders

- Usually, drug orders are recorded one of three ways:

  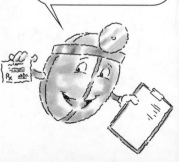 entering the order into a computer system that transmits to the pharmacy and nurses' station

   writing the order on an order sheet in the patient's chart

   faxing the order to the pharmacy.
- All drug orders must include essential information that follows standard guidelines and a specific sequence.

Written orders

- The prescriber must include all this information on the drug order:
  - date and time of order
  - name of prescribed drug
  - dosage form (in accepted measurement system)
  - route of administration
  - administration schedule
  - restrictions or specifications
  - prescriber's signature
  - registration number for controlled drug (if applicable).
- There are standard guidelines for writing drug orders:
  - Write the generic name of the drug in all lower-case letters.
  - Use a capital letter for the trade name (if one is provided).
  - Use capital letters for all abbreviations (if used).
- The standard sequence is drug name, dose, administra-

> See, everything's here on the drug order...in proper sequence and with the correct capitalization and punctuation!

tion route, and time and frequency of administration.

Military time

- Some health care facilities require that all orders are written in military time—based on a 24-hour system.
- To write single-digit time from 1:00 a.m. to 9:59 a.m., add a zero before the time and remove the colon (1:00 a.m. = 0100 hours).
- To write double-digit times from 10:00 a.m. to 12:59 p.m., remove the colon (12:30 p.m. = 1230 hours).

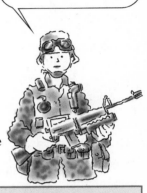

If you ask me, learning military time should warrant a gold star from the Surgeon General.

Writing in military time

Study these two clocks to better understand military time. The clock on the left represents the hours from 1 a.m. (0100 hours) to noon (1200 hours). The clock on the right represents the hours from 1 p.m. (1300 hours) to midnight (2400 hours).

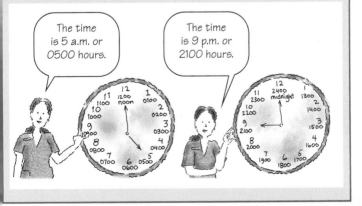

- The minutes after the hour remain the same (4:45 a.m. = 0445 hours).
- To write a time from 1:00 p.m. to 12 midnight, add 1200 to the number and remove the colon (3:35 p.m. = 1535 hours).
- To write times between 12:01 a.m. and 12:59 a.m., start over with zero (12:33 a.m. = 0033 hours).

Dealing with drug orders

- First, check the order for completeness; if information is missing, unclear, or illegible, clarify the order with the prescriber.
- Determine when to give the drug; although the drug order sheet will give the time of administration, the actual administration depends on three factors:

    facility policy (for drugs that are given a specific number of times per day)

    nature of the drug

    drug's onset and duration of action.

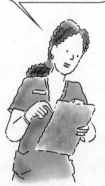

Check all drug orders for completeness, and document the precise time you administer drugs.

- Administer the drug within ½ hour of the time given on the drug order sheet; record the actual time of administration on the medication administration record (MAR).
- Follow facility policy for renewing all drug orders, including I.V. fluids; for example, opioids may need to be reordered every 24, 48, or 72 hours.
- If a drug needs to be discontinued before the original order runs out, make sure that the prescriber issues a new order to discontinue the drug.

Dodging drug dangers

Don't struggle with difficult orders

The combination of poor handwriting and inappropriate abbreviations on a drug order can lead to confusion and medication errors. Ask the prescriber to clarify an order that's difficult to understand or one that seems wrong.

FREEDOM HOSPITAL

UNIT NO. 4 SOUTH , 432A
NAME   JOE JACKSON
ADDRESS 33 SHORT STREET
CITY   HOPE , NJ BIRTH 2·21·24

DOCTOR'S ORDERS
INSTRUCTIONS
1. Each time a physicians writes a medication order, detach top copy and send to pharmacy.
2. Rule off unused lines after last copy (Pink) has been sent to pharmacy.

DO NOT USE THIS SHEET
UNLESS A NUMBER SHOWS.   **1**

DATE	TIME	ORDERS	DOCTOR'S SIGNATURE	NURSE'S SIGNATURE
2/14/07	12³⁰	*Beumt 2⁶/250 ? po @*		
		Captin 1g PO 340		
		Benadryl 25 mg PO HS		
		ROM exercise to all extremities		
		Soft diet patient mani chew		
		PD jm HD	D. Adams RN	
6/29/07		*DC Clonin*		
		DC Vancomycin		
		Kefzol 1.0 g IM q 6h		
		V Sentongin te 60 mg IV q 8 hrs		
6/30/07		*V Sentongin te 60 mg IV q 12h*		

Discharge diagnoses in order of decreasing priority must be supplied at time of patient's discharge.

Say it in English

These examples illustrate how to read and interpret several drug orders.

Drug order	Interpretation
Colace 100 mg P.O. b.i.d. p.c.	Give 100 mg of Colace by mouth twice per day after meals.
Vistaril 25 mg I.M. q3h p.r.n. anxiety	Give 25 mg of Vistaril intramuscularly every 3 hours as needed for anxiety.
Increase Duramorph to 6 mg I.V. q8h	Increase Duramorph to 6 mg intravenously every 8 hours.
folic acid 1 mg P.O. daily	Give 1 mg of folic acid by mouth daily.
Minipress 4 mg P.O. q6h, hold for sys BP < 120	Give 4 mg of Minipress by mouth every 6 hours; withhold the drug if the systolic blood pressure falls below 120 mm Hg.
nifedipine 30 mg S.L. q4h	Give 30 mg of nifedipine sublingually every 4 hours.
Begin aspirin 325 mg P.O. daily	Begin giving 325 mg of aspirin by mouth daily.
Persantine 75 mg P.O. t.i.d.	Give 75 mg of Persantine by mouth three times per day.
aspirin grains v P.O. t.i.d.	Give 5 grains of aspirin by mouth three times per day.
Vasotec 2.5 mg P.O. daily	Give 2.5 mg of Vasotec by mouth daily.
1,000 ml D_5W c̄ KCl 20 mEq I.V. at 100 ml/hr	Give 1,000 ml of dextrose 5% in water with 20 milliequivalents of potassium chloride intravenously at a rate of 100 milliliters per hour.
D/C penicillin I.V., start penicillin G 800,000 units P.O. q6h	Discontinue intravenous penicillin; start 800,000 units of penicillin G by mouth every 6 hours.
diphenhydramine 25-50 mg P.O. at bedtime p.r.n. insomnia	Give 25 to 50 mg of diphenhydramine by mouth at bedtime as needed for insomnia.

Knowing your responsibilities

- Make sure that the ordered drug is an appropriate treatment for the patient; use your critical-thinking skills.
- Know the action of each drug, why it's given, and its possible adverse effects.
- Know the patient; stay aware of allergies or other conditions that may affect or interfere with the drug's action.
- Always check a questionable drug order.
- Always check the five "rights" before giving a drug.

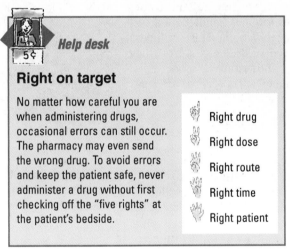

Help desk

Right on target

No matter how careful you are when administering drugs, occasional errors can still occur. The pharmacy may even send the wrong drug. To avoid errors and keep the patient safe, never administer a drug without first checking off the "five rights" at the patient's bedside.

- Right drug
- Right dose
- Right route
- Right time
- Right patient

- Check and recheck drug calculations carefully.
- Never administer an unlabeled drug or use open or unmarked I.V. bags.

Administration records

- Two main types of medication record systems are used in most facilities:

    ☝ the MAR—a paper form that goes into the patient's chart

    ✌ computer charting, which generates a list of administration times for all scheduled medications; this method also reduces the risk of drug errors from illegible handwriting.

- All medication records are legal documents.

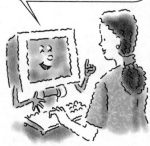

> Remember, I'm reliable but not infallible! You're still responsible for checking all orders carefully before administering drugs to patients.

Transcribing orders

- Transcription is necessary for MAR systems but not when computer systems are used.
- Before transcribing an order, make sure that the order is complete, clear, and correct; if any part is unclear, contact the prescriber.
- Use blue or black ink for clear reproduction, and write legibly.
- Begin by recording the patient's full name, identification number, unit number, bed

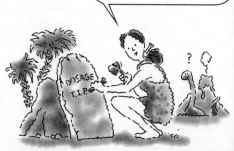

> Maybe someday, in the not-too-distant future, someone will invent an easier way to transcribe drug orders...this is exhausting, not to mention back-breaking!

Record keeping in the computer age

As health care facilities purchase or develop computer systems, manufacturers offer increased choices among medication monitoring programs. Computerized record systems range from simple to sophisticated.

From simple...
In the simplest systems, the computer is used as a word processor or typewriter.

...to sophisticated
In more sophisticated systems, prescribers can order drugs from the pharmacy by typing the drug's name, or they can select specific drugs by searching through various listings, such as pharmacologic categories, pharmacokinetic categories, and disease-related uses.

The computer indicates whether the pharmacy has the drug. The order then goes into the pharmacy's computer for filling. The order also generates a copy of the patient's record, on which the nurse can document medication administration. In some cases, the nurse can document medication administration on the computer.

Benefits bit by bit
Computer systems offer some advantages:
• When drug orders are changed, the pharmacy receives immediate notification, so drugs arrive on the unit faster.
• The pharmacy's computer can immediately confirm or deny a drug's availability.
• Nurses can document on medication administration records quickly and easily.
• Nurses can see at a glance which drugs have been administered and which still must be given.
• Errors from misinterpreted handwriting are eliminated.
• Records can be stored on disk in addition to—or instead of—paper copies.

number, and allergies on the MAR (write "NKA" if the patient has no known allergies).

What to document
• Here's what else you need to record:
  – date the order was written

Different forms, same info

This medication administration record illustrates the kind of information required on all types of medication administration forms. Although different facilities may use different forms, virtually all require the patient information, date, drug information, time of administration, and nurse's initials after administering the drug.

INITIAL	SIGNATURE	INITIAL	SIGNATURE
SA	Sally Adams RN		
JJ	Joan Johnson RN		

R = REFUSED O = OMITTED F = FASTING

JOE JACKSON
33 SHORT STREET
HOPE N.J   2·21·24
UNIT : 4 SOUTH 432 A

ALLERGIES
NKA

ROUTINE MEDICATIONS

DATE ORD.	STOP DATE	MEDICATION DOSE ROUTE FREQUENCY	R.N. INT.	HR.	2/14	2/15	2/16	2/17	2/18	2/19
2/14/07	2/19/07	carbidopa/levodopa (SINEMET) 25/250 P.O. Q.I.D	SA	A 10	X					
				P 2						
				P 6						
				P 10						
2/14/07	2/19/07	benztropine mesylate (COGENTIN) 1.0 mg P.O. T.I.D.	SA	A 10	X					
				P 2						
				P 6						
2/14/07	2/16/07	diphenhydramine hydrochloride (BENADRYL) 25 mg. P.O. H.S.	SA	P 10						

FREEDOM HOSPITAL

DIAGNOSIS & SURGERY   AGE   SEX   PHYSICIAN   ROOM   NAME

– date the drug should begin and stop (if known)
– drug's full generic name; if the trade name was used by the prescriber, record that as well (*Remember:* Don't use abbreviations, chemical symbols, research names, or other unapproved names.)
– amount of drug to be administered; if the amount administered varies from the amount ordered, document the amount given and why
– dosage form ordered; make sure that the dosage form is appropriate for the patient
– route of administration; if a parenteral route is used, document the injection site as well
– administration schedule; include the dosage schedule (such as t.i.d. or q6h), and then translate this into actual time (using a 24-hour clock). (Most facilities have set administration times for giving drugs, so check your facility's policy.)

• Transcribe the order in the correct place on the MAR. *(Note:* Many facilities have special administration records for as-needed or one-time drugs, I.V. fluids, and controlled substances, so make sure that you're documenting on the right form.)

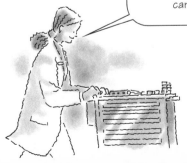

Keep in mind that you're administering drugs, not running a marathon. Take time to get to know your patient and make sure that you document carefully.

When and where to sign

- Always sign the MAR after transcribing the prescriber's order. Include your full name, title, and initials in the MAR's signature section; this same information must appear on every record you initial when administering drugs.
- If your facility requires you to perform a chart check (to make sure that all orders have been correctly transcribed onto the MAR), write your initials on the prescriber's order sheet on a line after the last order.

Recording what you administer

- Immediately after giving a drug, document that you administered the drug and the time it was given.
- If you don't give the exact amount of drug stipulated in the transcribed order, document the amount given and the reason why.
- If you don't give the drug on time or if you miss a dose, document the actual time the drug was given and the reason for the delay.
- If a parenteral route was used, document the specific site.
- Initial your entry on the MAR sheet (to make sure that another nurse doesn't repeat the same dose).

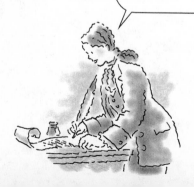

Putting your John Hancock on a medication administration record is serious business!

Drug errors

- Despite the best intentions, drug errors—some minor, some very serious—occur.
- Each member of the health care team has a responsibility for avoiding errors.
  – The prescriber (usually a doctor or other specially trained medical professional) must choose the right medication and write the order correctly.

  > We're all on the same team when it comes to medication administration.

  – The pharmacist must interpret the order, decide if it's complete, and correctly prepare and dispense the medication.
  – The nurse must evaluate whether the medication is appropriate for the patient and administer it correctly.
- Always follow your facility's policy on how and when to administer drugs to help prevent drug errors, and report all errors promptly.
- Know your responsibilities and be aware of your legal rights.

Types of errors

- Dosage calculation errors are the most common type of reported drug errors.
- Other errors may be common:
  – drug name errors
  – patient name errors
  – missed allergy alerts

Common drug errors

Certain situations or activities can place nurses at high risk for making a drug error. Some of the most common types and causes of errors are highlighted here.

Types of errors
- Giving the wrong drug
- Giving the wrong dose
- Using the wrong diluent
- Preparing the wrong concentration
- Missing a dose or failing to give an ordered drug
- Giving the drug at the wrong time
- Administering a drug to which the patient is allergic
- Infusing the drug too rapidly
- Giving the drug to the wrong patient
- Administering the drug by the wrong route

Causes
- Insufficient knowledge
- Chaotic work environment
- Use of floor stock medications
- Failure to follow facility policies and procedures

- Incorrect preparation or administration techniques
- Use of I.V. solutions that aren't premixed
- Failure to verify drug and dosage instructions
- Following oral, not written, orders
- Inadequate staffing
- Typographical errors
- Use of acronyms or erroneous abbreviations
- Math errors
- Poor handwriting
- Failure to check dosages for high-risk drugs or pediatric medications

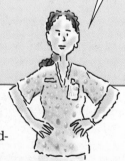

Unfortunately, drug errors can occur for many different reasons, so it's critical to take steps to prevent them.

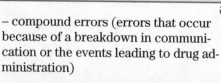

– compound errors (errors that occur because of a breakdown in communication or the events leading to drug administration)

Dodging drug dangers

Look-alike and sound-alike drug names

These drug names resemble each other in terms of spelling or sound. Always double-check the medication order carefully before administering one of them to your patient. If you have doubt about the appropriateness of the drug, consult the prescriber, the pharmacist, or a drug reference.

- amantadine and rimantadine
- amiodarone and amiloride
- amoxicillin and amoxapine
- benztropine and bromocriptine
- calcifediol and calcitriol
- Celebrex and Celexa
- cimetidine and simethicone
- codeine and Cardene
- Compazine and Thorazine
- desmopressin and vasopressin
- dexamethasone and desoximetasone
- digoxin and doxepin
- epinephrine and norepinephrine
- flunisolide and fluocinonide
- hydromorphone and morphine
- imipramine and desipramine
- Imuran and Inderal
- levothyroxine and liothyronine
- naloxone and naltrexone
- nifedipine and nicardipine
- nitroglycerin and nitroprusside
- pentobarbital and phenobarbital
- Ritalin and Rifadin
- sulfisoxazole and sulfasalazine
- vinblastine and vincristine
- Xanax and Zantac
- Zyrtec and Zyprexa

– drug route errors
– misinterpreted abbreviations
– misinterpreted orders
– preparation errors
– stress-related errors.

How to prevent errors

- Check drug orders carefully.
  – If a drug doesn't seem right or if you're unsure which drug is being ordered, ask the prescriber to clarify the order.

– Use all available resources (including consulting the pharmacist or a drug reference) to find out information about a new or unfamiliar drug.

> Consult the prescriber, not a crystal ball, when drug orders are vague, ambiguous, or confusing.

• Check the patient's identification carefully.
  – Be aware that patients may have the same or similar names, so always check the patient's full name and ask for an additional identifier such as his birth date.
  – Check the information against the MAR you bring into the room with you, and then check the MAR against the patient's hospital identification bracelet.
• Check the patient's allergies.
  – Check for allergies listed on the patient's chart, and ask the patient directly about allergies.

> You say your name is Grandma? Funny...you seem a tad hairier than I remember. Let me check your ID bracelet.

  – Be aware of the potential for cross-allergies; for example, patients who are allergic to sulfa drugs shouldn't receive certain hypoglycemic agents or certain diuretics.
  – Also ask about food allergies (certain medications shouldn't be given to patients with certain food allergies); for example, ipratropium given by metered-dose inhaler to someone with a peanut or soy allergy may cause anaphylaxis.
• Always administer the drug via the correct route.

– Most errors occur when a patient has several different lines running.
– One common mistake is giving an oral dose into a central I.V. line; be sure to prepare oral medications (including those to go through feeding tubes) in a syringe with a tip that's too large to fit in I.V. tubing.
– To help prevent giving an overdose through an I.V. line, never increase the drip rate to clear bubbles from the line; instead, remove the tubing from the pump, disconnect it from the patient, and use the flow-control clamp to purge the air.

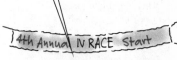

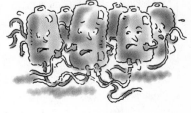

- Use and interpret abbreviations correctly.
  – Never abbreviate medications; always spell out all drug names.
  – Always clarify questionable medication orders.
  – Never use abbreviations that are known to increase the risk of drug errors. (A "Do not use" list should be posted on your unit.)

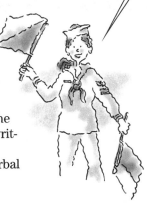

- Always double-check a phone or verbal order, and read it back to the prescriber to make sure that it's written correctly.
  – Follow all facility policies on verbal and phone orders.

JCAHO's "Do not use" list

All health care facilities accredited by the Joint Commission on Accreditation of Healthcare Organizations (JCAHO) are required to maintain a "Do not use" list—a list of abbreviations that should never be used in any form (upper or lower case, with or without periods) in clinical documentation because they're confusing and subject to misinterpretation.

Facilities are expected to include all of the abbreviations in the "Minimum required list" as well as at least three more from the "Additional recommended list" to remain compliant with JCAHO regulations.

Minimum required list
These abbreviations must appear on a "Do not use" list and should be avoided in all situations.

Abbreviation	Potential problem	Preferred term
U (for unit)	Mistaken as 0 (zero), 4 (four), or cc	Write *unit*.
IU (for international unit)	Mistaken as I.V. (intravenous) or 10 (ten)	Write *international unit*.
Q.D., QD, q.d., qd (daily); Q.O.D., QOD, q.o.d., qod (every other day)	Mistaken for each other (the period after the *Q* may be mistaken for an *I*, and the *O* may be mistaken for an *I*)	Write *daily* and *every other day*.
Trailing zero (as in *X.0 mg*), absence of leading zero (as in *.X mg*)	Inaccuracies with numbers or values due to missed decimal point	Never write a zero by itself after a decimal point *(X mg)*, and always use a zero before a decimal point *(0.X mg)*.

JCAHO's "Do not use" list *(continued)*

Additional recommended abbreviations

Facilities are expected to add at least three of these abbreviations to their "Do not use" list, in addition to those included in the "Minimum required list." They're encouraged to expand the list as needed.

Abbreviation	Potential problem	Preferred term
MS, MSO_4, $MgSO_4$	Confused for one another (can mean morphine sulfate or magnesium sulfate)	Write *morphine sulfate* or *magnesium sulfate*.
µg (for microgram)	Mistaken for mg (milligrams), resulting in a thousandfold overdose	Write *mcg*.
cc (for cubic centimeter)	Mistaken for *U* (units) when poorly written	Write *ml* for *milliliters*.
> (greater than) < (less than)	Misinterpreted as the number *7* (seven) or the letter *L*; confused for one another	Write *greater than.* Write *less than.*
Drug name abbreviations	Misinterpreted due to similar abbreviations for multiple drugs	Write drug names in full.
Apothecary units	Unfamiliar to many practitioners; confused with metric units	Use metric units.
@	Mistaken for the number *2* (two)	Write *at.*

  – Have the prescriber sign the order as soon as possible after transcribing it.
- Always check the drug's appearance before administering it, and only administer a drug that you've personally prepared.
  – If a drug is unfamiliar or seems unusual (such as discolored, cloudy, or too concentrated), verify that it's the correct drug.

– Check for unusual odors.
– Never give a drug that has no label or that has an ambiguous or incorrect label.

- Always return unused or discontinued medications to the pharmacy.
- Teach the patient about the drugs he's taking—what they look like, how they're given, and when he should receive them. Encourage him to question unfamiliar medications.
- Take appropriate steps to reduce stress.

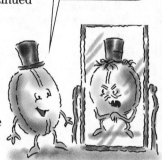

I can't put my finger on it, but something's off...I just don't seem the same today.

Preventing drug errors through teaching

Drug errors aren't limited to hospital settings. Patients sometimes make drug errors when taking their medications at home. To prevent such errors, take the time to educate your patient thoroughly about each medication he'll be taking. Be sure to cover these points:
- drug's name (generic and trade name)
- drug's purpose
- correct dosage and how to calculate it (such as breaking scored tablets or mixing liquids when necessary)
- how to take the drug
- when to take the drug
- what to do if a dose is missed
- how to monitor the drug's effectiveness (for example, checking blood glucose level when taking a hypoglycemic drug)
- potential drug interactions (including the need to avoid certain over-the-counter and herbal drugs)
- required dietary changes (including the use of alcohol)
- possible adverse effects and what to do if they occur
- proper storage, handling, and disposal of the drug or supplies (such as syringes)
- required follow-up.

Dodging drug dangers

Conquering confusion

Before giving a drug, take a moment to remind yourself of these essential tactics.

Remember the five rights.
Check that you're giving the right drug, at the right dose, by the right route, at the right time, and to the right patient.

Double-check the math.
You can never be too safe. Go over your math at least twice to make sure that your calculations are correct.

Look at the label.
Examine drug labels closely—many of them look alike.

Notice the name.
Pay attention! Many drugs have similar-sounding or similar-looking names.

– Many drug errors occur because nurses are in a hurry or under a great deal of stress.
– Try to take your time, avoid distractions, and seek help from colleagues to minimize errors.

Refusing to give a drug

- A nurse may legally refuse to give a drug under certain conditions:
  – the prescribed dosage is too high
  – the drug might interact dangerously with other drugs the patient is taking
  – the patient's physical condition contraindicates use of the drug.
- If you refuse to give a drug, notify the prescriber and document why the drug wasn't given.

Documenting and tracking drug errors

- Follow your facility's policy for reporting and tracking drug errors.
  - All errors must be reported through the proper channels.
  - Quality assurance teams review errors and examine procedures to help prevent future episodes, not to place blame; safety precautions and performance improvement recommendations can also help prevent errors.
- If you make an error, report the incident promptly.
  - Notify the prescriber immediately.
  - Consult the pharmacist about possible drug interactions, solutions to dose-related problems, and whether an antidote is available (if needed).
  - Continue to monitor the patient's condition.
  - Document the error according to your facility's policy, including filing an incident report (if necessary).

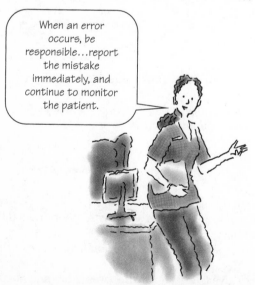

Oral, topical, and rectal drugs

4

Grab your suitcase and road atlas...we'll be covering a lot of ground and a few different routes—oral, topical, and rectal—on this trip. And, if there's enough time, we'll even swing by Route 66...just for kicks, of course!

Administering oral drugs

- Oral drugs are usually administered in tablet, capsule, or liquid form.
- Most oral drugs are available in a limited number of strengths or concentrations, so knowing how to calculate dosages is important.
- In some cases, you'll need to administer an oral analgesic in place of a parenteral (injectable) analgesic; this requires a conversion using an equianalgesic chart.

Read the label

- Before administering a drug, make sure it's the right drug and the right dose.
- Check the label carefully, paying special attention to:
  - drug name
  - dose strength
  - expiration date.

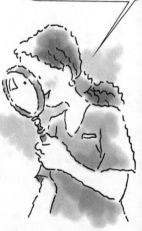

Look closely! All the essential information about giving a drug should be right on the label.

Drug name

- Always check the generic name first.
  - All drugs have a generic name.
  - The name is typically in lowercase print; it may be in parentheses.
  - It should appear under the trade name.
- Next check the trade (brand, or proprietary) name.
  - Not all drugs have a trade name (for example, atropine sulfate doesn't have a trade name).
  - The first letter is generally capitalized; it's usually followed by a registration (®) symbol.

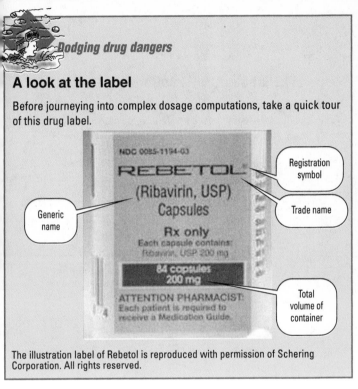

- Some oral medications are a combination of two drugs.
  - The generic names and doses of both drugs are listed on the label.
  - The prescriber commonly orders a combination medication by its trade name.

Dose strength
- Always check the drug strength on the label.
- Many drugs come in different concentrations. In most cases, the packaging for different concentrations will be exactly the same—except for the dose strength listed on the label; so, it's important to read all labels closely.

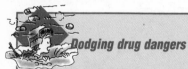

Dodging drug dangers

Look-alike labels: Oral solutions

The oral solution labels below are examples of look-alikes that you're likely to encounter. Reading labels carefully can help you avoid medication errors.

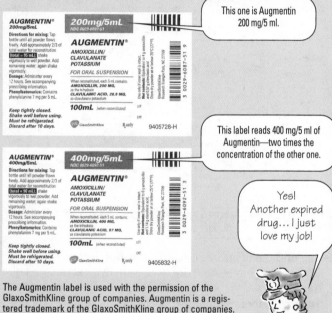

This one is Augmentin 200 mg/5 ml.

This label reads 400 mg/5 ml of Augmentin—two times the concentration of the other one.

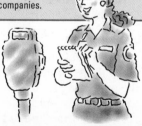

Yes! Another expired drug... I just love my job!

The Augmentin label is used with the permission of the GlaxoSmithKline group of companies. Augmentin is a registered trademark of the GlaxoSmithKline group of companies.

Expiration date

• Expired drugs may be unstable or may not provide the correct dose.

• Return all expired drugs to the pharmacy.

Check, double-check, and triple-check

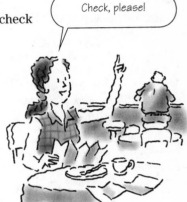

Check, please!

• Before giving a drug, always check the five rights:

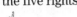 Right drug

Right route

Right dose

Right time

Right patient.

• Then triple-check the drug label against the drug order, following these essential steps, before administering the drug:
  – Obtain the drug from the medication supply (drawer, shelf, or cabinet).
  – Check the drug name and dose, and make sure it's in the correct oral form *(First check)*.
  – Place the labeled drug next to the transcribed order on the administration record, and compare each part of the label with the order *(Second check)*.
  – If taking a drug from a bulk or stock bottle, transfer the appropriate number of tablets from the supply into a medication container without handling the tablets. If giving a liquid medication, measure carefully with a calibrated medicine cup, dropper, or syringe.

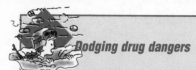

Dodging drug dangers

Say it three times: Check orders and labels

The secret of drug safety is to check, check, and check again. Before giving a drug, carefully compare the drug's label with each part of the medication administration record, holding the label next to the administration record to ensure accuracy. The example below walks you through the steps for administering *furosemide (Lasix) 40 mg P.O.*

Check drug names.
• Read the drug's generic name on the administration record and compare it with the generic name on the label. They both should read *furosemide*.
• Read the trade name on the administration record and compare it with the trade name on the label. They both should read *Lasix*.

Check the dosage, route, and record.
• Read the dosage on the administration record and compare it with the dose on the label. They both should read *40 mg.*
• Read the route specified on the administration record and note the dose form on the label. The record should read *P.O.,* and the label should read *oral tablet.*
• Note any special considerations on the administration record, such as "aspiration precautions (head of bed elevated to 45 degrees for all P.O. intake)," "Patient is HOH (hard of hearing)," or "Patient is blind."

Check orders and labels three times.
Follow this routine three times before giving the drug. Do it the first time when you obtain the drug from floor stock or from the patient's supply. Do it the second time before placing the drug in the medication cup or other administration device. Lastly, do it the third time before replacing the stock drug bottle on the shelf or removing the drug from the unit-dose package at the patient's bedside.

- Before returning the supply to the drawer or shelf, compare the label with the order on the administration record, and make sure it's the right time to administer the drug.
- Next, go to the patient's bedside, check the identification bracelet, and check the drug one more time *(Third check)*. If all the information matches, administer the drug.
- If the drug comes in a unit-dose pack, don't remove the drug from the packet until you're at the patient's beside and ready to administer the drug (do your third check then). Remove the drug from the packet and give it to the patient;

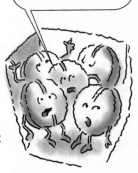

use the packet label for comparison when recording your administration information.

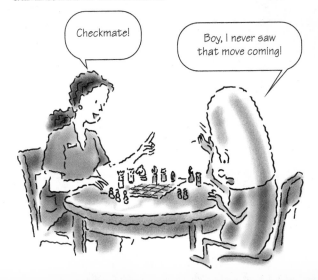

- Investigate discrepancies between the medication administration record and the drug label.
  - Consult a reliable source (pharmacist or a drug handbook) if you note any differences.
  - Perform needed dosage calculations.

Measure carefully

- Many oral drugs are available in tablet or capsule form and need to be counted (in some cases, scored and split) before giving them to the patient.
- Many drugs are also prepackaged in unit doses, eliminating the need for measurement.

Unit-dose packaging

Tablets or capsules in unit doses may be dispensed on a card with the drugs sealed in bubbles or in strips with each drug separated by a tear line. Unit doses of liquids may be packaged in small sealed cups with identifying information on the cover.

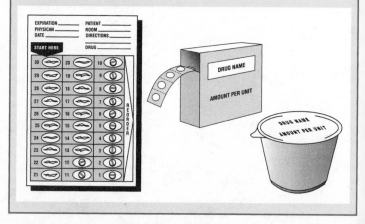

- Many drugs are prepared and administered as oral solutions; some are in powder form and need to be diluted in a solution before you can administer them.
- In some situations, you'll need to substitute an oral analgesic for an injectable one for pain control; this requires special calculations.

Measuring oral solutions

- To ensure accurate measurement of an oral solution, always use a medicine cup, dropper, or syringe.
- Medicine cups are calibrated to measure in milliliters, tablespoons, teaspoons, drams, and ounces.
  - Hold the cup at eye level while pouring the solution.
  - Hold the solution container with the medication label turned toward your palm to prevent the solution from dripping on the label when poured.

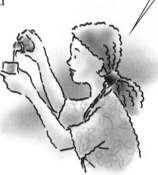

As with everything, it's all in the technique. Hold the cup at eye level, watch for drips, and pour with a steady hand.

- Drugs that are prescribed in drops are usually packaged with a dropper; droppers measure solutions in milliliters or teaspoons.
- Syringes are used to draw up and accurately measure solutions; they shouldn't be used to administer an oral drug.

Diluting powders

- Some drugs become unstable when stored as liquids and are supplied in powder form.
- Always read the drug label to see how much and what diluent to use to dilute the powder.
- Be sure to mix thoroughly after adding the diluent.
- The dose concentration in oral solutions is expressed as the weight (dose strength) of the drug in a volume of solution (usually milliliters).

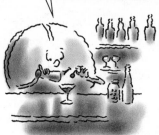

A special order for the patient in room 007—he likes his oral medications shaken, not stirred!

Splitting scored tablets

- In some cases, you may need to break a tablet to give a smaller dose.
- Only break scored tablets.
- If a tablet is unscored (or if it must be broken into a portion smaller than one-half), substitute a commercially available solution or suspension or ask the pharmacist to prepare one.
- Most tablets shouldn't be broken into portions smaller than one-half because the dose may be inaccurate.
- Be aware that not all oral medications can be scored or broken.

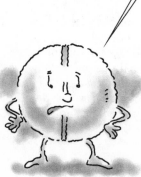

At least with me, I know where the ax will fall... I just don't have a clue when.

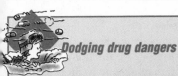

Dodging drug dangers

Dividing tablets and capsules

Before you break or crush a tablet or capsule, call the pharmacist to see if the drug is available in smaller dosage strengths or in liquid form for patients who have difficulty swallowing. Also check your drug handbook—or check with the pharmacist—to see if altering the drug will affect its action. Drugs that shouldn't be broken or crushed include:

• sustained-release drugs, also called *extended-release, timed-release,* or *controlled-release* (Suffixes such as "SR," "CR," "DUR," and "LA" in a drug name usually indicate that the drug is sustained-release.)

• capsules that contain tiny beads of medication, although you may empty the contents of some of these capsules into a beverage, pudding, or applesauce

• enteric-coated tablets, which have a hard coating (usually shiny or glossy) that's designed to protect the upper GI tract from irritation

• buccal and sublingual tablets.

Tips for crushing and breaking

If you need to crush a tablet, use a chewable form, which is softer. The easiest method is to crush the tablet while it's still in its package, using a hemostat or pill crusher. Or, you can remove it from the package and crush it with a mortar and pestle.

If you need to break a tablet, use one that's scored. Carefully cut the tablet on the score line with a pill cutter. Enlist the pharmacist's help when you need to break a tablet into smaller pieces than the score allows or when you must administer a portion of a capsule. If you need to break an unscored tablet, have the pharmacist crush, weigh, and dispense it in two equal doses.

Substituting equianalgesic drugs

- At times, you may need to administer an oral analgesic (pain medication) in place of a parenteral (I.M. injected) drug.
- To convert a parenteral dose of an analgesic to an oral dose, use an equianalgesic chart.

Equianalgesic charts: A painless path for converting dosages

When substituting one analgesic for another, equianalgesic charts provide the information you need to calculate the dose necessary to produce the desired pain control (equianalgesic effect).

These charts use morphine sulfate as the *gold standard* for comparison. On most charts, doses for many drugs are listed; each dose provides pain relief equivalent to 10 mg of I.M. morphine. Here's an example of an equianalgesic chart.

Medication	I.M. dose	P.O. dose
Morphine	10 mg	30 mg
Codeine	1.5 mg	7.5 mg
Hydromorphone	2 mg	4 mg
Levorphanol	130 mg	200 mg
Meperidine	75 mg	300 mg

Remember: Every dose on the equianalgesic chart provides an equivalent amount of pain control, and any change in medication requires a prescriber's order.

Calculating oral tablet dosages

- Even with unit-dose systems, you'll still need to make dosage calculations in order to administer many oral drugs.

Help desk

Special-delivery drug dosages

Even if your facility uses the unit-dose system, you'll still need to calculate dosages for some patients. For example, patients on intensive care units, pediatric patients, and geriatric patients require individualized medication dosages that may be unusually large or small.

The nearest milligram
Some patients need doses that are calculated to the nearest milligram instead of the nearest 10 mg. For them, the correct calculation of the exact dose can mean the difference between an underdose or overdose and the correct dose. A few examples of drugs that are measured to the nearest milligram or microgram are digoxin, levothyroxine sodium, and many pediatric drugs.

Changing the delivery route
Some people can't handle drugs that are delivered by the usual route because their ability to absorb, distribute, metabolize, or excrete drugs is impaired. Some patients can't absorb drugs from the GI tract because of upper GI disorders or surgery; deficiencies of gastric, pancreatic, or intestinal secretions; or passive congestion of GI blood vessels from severe heart failure. These patients need drugs in parenteral form in larger-than-average oral doses. Smaller doses of a drug can be used when the drug is given I.V. because it may be delivered to the bloodstream more efficiently and is more readily absorbed.

Don't forget these special patients
Other patients who need individualized doses include those with conditions that cause abnormal drug distribution from the GI tract or from parenteral sites to the sites of action. Premature infants and patients with low serum

(continued)

Special-delivery drug dosages *(continued)*

protein levels or severe liver or kidney disease who can't metabolize or excrete drugs as readily as normal patients also require special drug dosages. You can help individualize drug regimens for these patients by assessing their kidney or liver function, monitoring blood levels of drugs, and calculating exact dosages.

- In many cases, you'll need to convert between measurement systems.
- Follow these four rules to simplify your calculations and help prevent medication and math errors:

  Make sure you're using the correct units of measure.

  Double-check decimals and zeros.

  Question any strange answers you get.

  Always use a calculator.

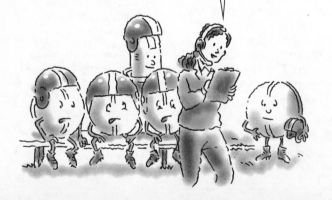

Help desk

Helpful hints to minimize math mistakes

To avoid math mistakes when computing dosages, use these helpful hints:

• Write out all calculations, using the proper formula.
• Recheck your calculations with another nurse or the pharmacist.

Use correct units of measure

• Using incorrect units of measure is one of the most common calculation errors.
• Remember to match units of measure in the numerator and denominator to cancel the units out; this leaves the correct unit of measure.

Learn by example

How many milligrams of a drug are in two tablets if one tablet contains 5 mg of the drug?

• State the problem as a proportion:

  $$5 \text{ mg} : 1 \text{ tablet} :: X : 2 \text{ tablets}$$

• Remember the product of the means equals the product of the extremes:

  $$1 \text{ tablet} \times X = 5 \text{ mg} \times 2 \text{ tablets}$$

• Solve for X. Divide each side of the equation by the known value, 1 tablet, and cancel units that appear in both the numerator and denominator:

  $$\frac{\cancel{1 \text{ tablet}} \times X}{\cancel{1 \text{ tablet}}} = \frac{5 \text{ mg} \times 2 \cancel{\text{ tablets}}}{1 \cancel{\text{ tablet}}}$$

  $$X = 10 \text{ mg}$$

> Make sure you're using the right units, and set up your equation so that "like" units cancel out.

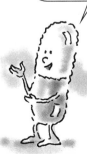

Double-check decimals and zeros

- A decimal place error can cause a tenfold or greater dosage error.
- A missing or misplaced zero can also have disastrous effects.

Learn by example

A patient is scheduled to receive 0.05 mg levothyroxine P.O., but the only drug on hand is in tablets that contain 0.025 mg each. How many tablets should you give?

- State the problem as a proportion:

    0.025 mg : 1 tablet :: 0.05 mg : X

- The product of the means equals the product of the extremes:

    1 tablet × 0.05 mg = 0.025 mg × X

- Solve for X by dividing each side of the equation by 0.025 mg and canceling units that appear in both the numerator and denominator. Carefully check the decimal placement.

$$\frac{1 \text{ tablet} \times 0.05 \text{ mg}}{0.025 \text{ mg}} = \frac{0.025 \text{ mg} \times X}{0.025 \text{ mg}}$$

$$X = 2 \text{ tablets}$$

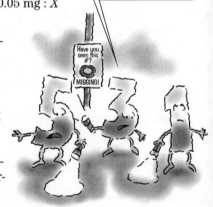

Everyone spread out and check the perimeter... he's big and round, and he may be wearing a small decimal point.

Have you seen this #?

MISSING!

Question strange answers
- Always recheck calculations that result in suspicious-looking answers.
- If you're still unsure about the answer after checking, ask another nurse to check your calculation.

Use a calculator
- A calculator will usually improve the accuracy and speed of your calculations, but it can't set up proportions for you.
- Always double-check units of measure and decimal places.

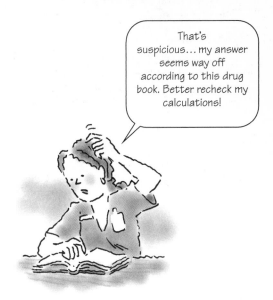

That's suspicious... my answer seems way off according to this drug book. Better recheck my calculations!

Calculating liquid dosages

- Before calculating a liquid dose, read the label carefully to identify the dose strength in a specified amount of solution; then check the label for the expiration date.
- Use a proportion to calculate the amount of solution needed.
  - Set up the first ratio or fraction with the known solution strength.
  - Set up the second ratio or fraction with the desired dose and the unknown quantity.
  - Then solve for X.

Learn by example

Your patient is receiving 500 mg of cefaclor in an oral suspension. The label reads 250 mg/5 ml, and the bottle contains 100 ml. How many milliliters of the drug should you give?

- First, set up the first fraction with the known solution strength:

$$\frac{5 \text{ ml}}{250 \text{ mg}}$$

- Next, set up the second fraction with the desired dose and the unknown number of milliliters:

$$\frac{X}{500 \text{ mg}}$$

- Now, put these numbers into a proportion:

$$\frac{X}{500 \text{ mg}} = \frac{5 \text{ ml}}{250 \text{ mg}}$$

- Cross-multiply the fractions:

$$X \times 250 \text{ mg} = 5 \text{ ml} \times 500 \text{ mg}$$

- Solve for X by dividing both sides of the equation by 250 mg and canceling units that appear in both the numerator and denominator:

$$\frac{X \times \cancel{250 \text{ mg}}}{\cancel{250 \text{ mg}}} = \frac{5 \text{ ml} \times 500 \cancel{\text{ mg}}}{250 \cancel{\text{ mg}}}$$

$$X = \frac{2,500 \text{ ml}}{250}$$

$$X = 10 \text{ ml}$$

- You'll need to administer 10 ml of cefaclor to the patient.

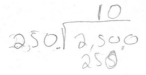

Performing two-step calculations

- Most dosage calculations require more than one equation.
- In many cases, you'll need to convert from one measurement system to another before determining the amount of medication to administer.
- To convert between two measurement systems, use a conversion chart to find the standard equivalent value.
  - Then use the ratio-and-proportion or fraction method to calculate the correct dose.
  - Put the standard equivalent values in the first ratio or fraction, and put the quantity ordered and the unknown quantity in the second ratio or fraction.

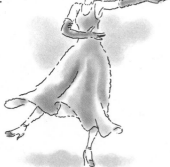

Sometimes that extra step makes all the difference!

Help desk

When you need a new measure

To easily determine a dose when you must first convert to a different measurement system, remember these tips:
- Read the drug order thoroughly, paying close attention to decimal places and zeros.
- Convert the dose from the system in which it's ordered to the system in which it's available.
- Calculate the number of capsules or tablets or the amount of solution needed to obtain the desired dose.

Learn by example

Your patient's order, written in apothecaries' units, reads *aspirin gr x P.O. daily*, but the unit-dose package says *aspirin 325 mg*. How many tablets should you administer daily?

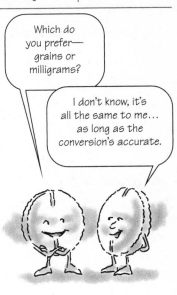

Step 1

- Remember that *aspirin gr x* means 10 grains of aspirin (1 grain is equivalent to approximately 65 mg).
- First, set up the first fraction with the standard equivalent values:

$$\frac{65 \text{ mg}}{1 \text{ grain}}$$

- Next, set up the second fraction with the unknown quantity in the appropriate position:

$$\frac{X}{10 \text{ grains}}$$

- Now, put these fractions into a proportion:

$$\frac{65 \text{ mg}}{1 \text{ grain}} = \frac{X}{10 \text{ grains}}$$

- Cross-multiply the fractions to set up an equation:

$$65 \text{ mg} \times 10 \text{ grains} = X \times 1 \text{ grain}$$

- Solve for X by dividing both sides of the equation by 1 grain and canceling units that appear in the numerator and denominator:

$$\frac{65 \text{ mg} \times 10 \text{ grains}}{1 \text{ grain}} = \frac{X \times 1 \text{ grain}}{1 \text{ grain}}$$

$$X = 650 \text{ mg}$$

- Now you know that you'll need to give the patient 650 mg.

Step 2

- To determine the number of tablets, you need to set up a proportion:

$$\frac{X}{650 \text{ mg}} = \frac{1 \text{ tablet}}{325 \text{ mg}}$$

- Cross-multiply the fractions:

$$X \times 325 \text{ mg} = 1 \text{ tablet} \times 650 \text{ mg}$$

- Solve for X by dividing each side of the equation by 325 mg and canceling units that appear in both the numerator and denominator:

$$\frac{X \times 325 \text{ mg}}{325 \text{ mg}} = \frac{1 \text{ tablet} \times 650 \text{ mg}}{325 \text{ mg}}$$

$$\frac{650 \text{ tablets}}{325 \text{ mg}}$$

$$X = 1\tfrac{4}{5} \text{ tablets}$$

- You should give the patient 2 tablets.

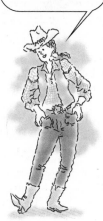

Here's where the old two-step comes in.

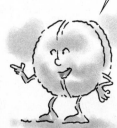

Remember, sometimes it's better to round off a dose when your answer contains a fraction or a very small portion.

Using the desired-over-have method

• Another way of solving two-step problems is the desired-over-have method, which uses fractions to express the known and unknown quantities in proportions:

$$\frac{\text{amount desired}}{\text{amount you have}} = \frac{\text{equivalent amount desired}}{\text{equivalent amount you have}}$$

• Make sure the units of measure in the numerator and denominator of the first fraction correspond to the units of measure in the numerator and denominator of the second fraction.

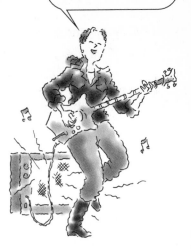

"You can't always get what you want..." Bet whoever wrote that one didn't know much about dosage calculations!

Learn by example

A drug order calls for 60 mEq potassium chloride liquid as a one-time dose, but the only solution on hand contains 20 mEq/15 ml. How many tablespoons should you give the patient?

• First convert the milliliters to tablespoons by using a conversion table. You'll see that 15 ml equals 1 tbs; therefore, 20 mEq of the solution on hand equals 1 tbs.

- Next, set up the first fraction with the amount desired over the amount you have:

$$\frac{60 \text{ mEq}}{20 \text{ mEq}}$$

- Now, set up the second fraction with the unknown amount desired—X—in the appropriate position:

$$\frac{X}{1 \text{ tbs}}$$

- Put these fractions into a proportion:

$$\frac{X \text{ desired}}{1 \text{ tbs have}} = \frac{60 \text{ mEq desired}}{20 \text{ mEq have}}$$

- Cross-multiply the fractions:

$$X \times 20 \text{ mEq} = 1 \text{ tbs} \times 60 \text{ mEq}$$

- Solve for X by dividing each side of the equation by 20 mEq and canceling units that appear in both the numerator and denominator:

$$\frac{X \times \cancel{20 \text{ mEq}}}{\cancel{20 \text{ mEq}}} = \frac{1 \text{ tbs} \times 60 \cancel{\text{ mEq}}}{20 \cancel{\text{ mEq}}}$$

$$X = 3 \text{ tbs}$$

- The patient should receive 3 tbs of potassium chloride liquid.

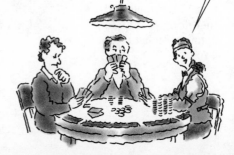

My idea of a conversion table is a dining room table that converts easily to a poker table. OK, ante-up, boys!

Topical and rectal drugs

- Drugs administered topically include:
  - creams
  - lotions
  - ointments
  - powders
  - patches.
- Topical drugs are applied to the skin and absorbed through the epidermis into the dermis; they're used for their local and systemic effects.
- Rectal drugs are used for patients who can't take drugs orally.
- Drugs administered rectally include:
  - enemas
  - suppositories.

Always wash your hands and follow your facility's protocol when administering any topical or rectal drug.

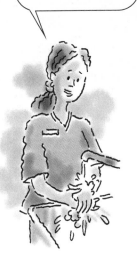

Read all labels

- Always read the label closely before using any topical or rectal drug.
- The trade name will appear first, then the generic name, dose strength, and total volume of the package.
- Some labels contain special administration information, so read carefully.

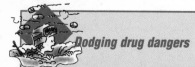

Dodging drug dangers

Labeling a successful administration

There are three rules for administering medication: Read the label, read the label, and read the label.

A topical topic

When reading a topical ointment label, note the information shown on this box label:

- generic name (mupirocin)
- trade name (Bactroban)
- dose strength (2% ointment)
- total package volume (22 grams)
- special instructions (not included on this label).

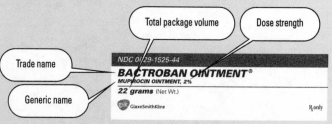

The Bactroban ointment label is used with the permission of the GlaxoSmithKline group of companies. Bactroban ointment is a registered trademark of the GlaxoSmithKline group of companies.

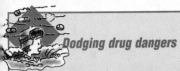

Dodging drug dangers

Combination product alert

Topical preparations may contain more than one drug. For example, Mycitracin Plus pain reliever ointment contains bacitracin, neomycin, polymyxin B, and lidocaine. Carefully note all ingredients when checking labels, and make sure that your patient isn't allergic to any of them.

Transdermal patches

- Transdermal patches administer drugs by passive diffusion at a constant rate.
- They're used to administer drugs that aren't well absorbed in the GI tract or that are metabolized and eliminated too quickly.
- Drug concentration in transdermal patches can vary based on the design of the patch.
  - Concentration of the drug isn't as important as the drug's rate of release.
  - Patches with different concentrations may release the drug at the same rate.

Prescribed patches

These transdermal drugs allow you to topically administer systemic drugs.

Nitroglycerin

Transdermal nitroglycerin provides prophylactic treatment of chronic angina. Available brands include Deponit, Nitrodisc, Nitro-Dur, and Transderm-Nitro. A new patch is applied daily (usually in the morning) and removed after 12 to 14 hours to prevent the patient from developing a tolerance to the drug.

Nicotine

Transdermal nicotine is used to treat smoking addiction. Brands include Habitrol, Nicoderm, Nicotrol, and ProStep. These drugs should be used only as adjuncts to behavioral therapy programs. A new patch is applied daily. Nicotrol should be removed after 16 hours, but other brands should stay on for 24 hours.

Fentanyl

Transdermal fentanyl is administered to treat severe chronic pain. Its brand name is Duragesic. Each patch may be worn up to 72 hours.

Clonidine

Clonidine is used to treat hypertension. The brand name for this drug is Catapres TTS. A new patch is applied every 7 days.

Scopolamine

Scopolamine is used to treat nausea, vomiting, and vertigo. Brands include Transderm-Scop. The patch is applied to the skin behind the ear at least 4 hours before an antiemetic effect is needed. It can be worn for 3 days.

Estradiol

Transdermal estradiol provides hormone replacement to estrogen-deficient women. The brand names include Climara, Estraderm, and Vivelle. It's administered on an intermittent cyclic schedule (3 weeks of therapy followed by discontinuation for 1 week).

Testosterone

Transdermal testosterone provides hormone replacement for men with testosterone deficiency. The brand names are Androderm and Testoderm. The Testoderm patch is applied once daily to clean, hairless scrotal skin, which is the only skin that's thin enough to allow adequate blood levels to be achieved.

Topical drug dosages

- Topical drug dosages typically require very little calculation.
- Transdermal patches are changed at regular intervals to ensure the patient receives the correct dose.
- When an ointment is prescribed, the prescriber should indicate how much to use.
  - The amount specified may be general such as "use a thin layer."
  - When used for a systemic effect, the administration guidelines are usually more specific.
- Ointments that come in a tube commonly have a paper ruler applicator to measure the correct dose.

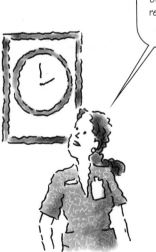

Patches eliminate the need for dosage calculations—a big plus. But they must be checked frequently and replaced according to a set schedule.

Measuring a topical dose

To measure a specified amount of ointment from a tube, squeeze the prescribed length of ointment in inches or centimeters onto a paper ruler like the one shown here. Then use the ruler to apply the ointment to the patient's skin at the appropriate time, following the manufacturer's guidelines for administration.

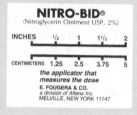

NITRO-BID®
(Nitroglycerin Ointment USP, 2%)

INCHES	½	1	1½	2

CENTIMETERS	1.25	2.5	3.75	5

the applicator that measures the dose

E. FOUGERA & CO.
a division of Altana Inc.
MELVILLE, NEW YORK 11747

Rectal drug dosages

- To calculate the number of suppositories to give, use the proportion method with ratios or fractions.
- The prescribed dose is typically one suppository, but two may be required.

Two suppositories may be required.

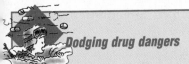

Dodging drug dangers

Check and check again

Occasionally you may need to insert more than one or a portion of one suppository. Here's what to do.

More than one
Do your dosage calculations indicate a need for more than one suppository? If so, check your figures and ask another nurse to check them, too. Then ask the pharmacist whether the suppository is available in other dosage strengths.

More than two
If more than two suppositories are needed, confirm the dose with the prescriber. Then check with the pharmacist. He may be able to give you one suppository with an adequate amount of the drug.

A portion of one
If less than one suppository is needed, check your calculations and have another nurse do the same. Then ask the pharmacist if the dose is available in one suppository. This ensures the most accurate dose.

Learn by example

Your pediatric patient needs 240 mg of acetaminophen by suppository. The package label reads acetaminophen suppositories 120 mg. How many suppositories should you give?

• Set up the first fraction with the known suppository dose:

$$\frac{1 \text{ supp}}{120 \text{ mg}}$$

- Set up the second fraction with the desired dose and the unknown number of suppositories:

$$\frac{X}{240 \text{ mg}}$$

- Put these fractions into a proportion:

$$\frac{1 \text{ supp}}{120 \text{ mg}} = \frac{X}{240 \text{ mg}}$$

- Cross-multiply the fractions:

$$120 \text{ mg} \times X = 1 \text{ supp} \times 240 \text{ mg}$$

- Solve for X by dividing each side of the equation by 120 mg and canceling units that appear in both the numerator and denominator:

$$\frac{\cancel{120 \text{ mg}} \times X}{\cancel{120 \text{ mg}}} = \frac{1 \text{ supp} \times 240 \cancel{\text{ mg}}}{120 \cancel{\text{ mg}}}$$

$$X = 2 \text{ suppositories}$$

- In this case, administer 2 suppositories.

Parenteral drugs

5

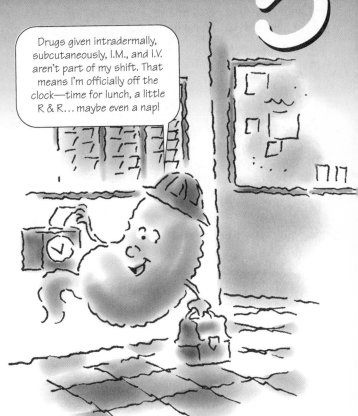

Drugs given intradermally, subcutaneously, I.M., and I.V. aren't part of my shift. That means I'm officially off the clock—time for lunch, a little R & R... maybe even a nap!

Administering drugs parenterally

- Parenteral drugs are administered through skin, subcutaneous tissue, muscle, or veins; they avoid the G.I. system (the term *parenteral* means "outside the intestines").
- They require calculations to determine the correct amount of liquid medication to inject.
- Four types of parenteral injections include:

  ✌ intradermal

  ✌ subcutaneous

  ✌ I.M.

  ✌ I.V. (discussed in the next chapter).

- To give an injection safely, you must be familiar with the specific injection sites, syringes, and needles used for each type of injection.

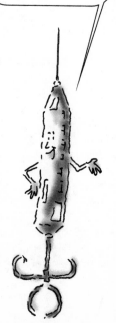

> I get your point—you need to stay sharp and focus on your technique to give a parenteral injection!

Intradermal injections

- Medication is injected into the dermis (outer layer of skin).
- Common uses for intradermal injections include anesthetizing skin for invasive procedures and testing for allergies, tuberculosis, histoplasmosis, and other diseases.
- The volume of a drug given intradermally is less than 0.5 ml.
- To give an injection, use a 1-ml syringe that's calibrated in 0.01-ml increments with a 25- to 27-gauge needle that's $3/8''$ to $5/8''$ long.

- There are four steps to performing an intradermal injection:

  Thoroughly clean the skin.

  Stretch the skin taut with one hand.

  With your other hand, quickly insert the needle at a 10- to 15-degree angle to a depth of about 0.5 cm.

  Inject the drug. A small wheal should form where the drug is injected.

Subcutaneous injections

- The drug is injected into the subcutaneous tissue, below the dermis and above the muscle.
- The drug is absorbed faster than in the dermis due to increased capillaries.
- Drugs commonly injected subcutaneously (subQ) include:
  – insulin
  – heparin
  – tetanus toxoid.
- A volume of 0.5 to 1 ml can be injected subQ.
- Needles used for subQ injections are 23G to 28G and $1/2''$ to $5/8''$ long.
- Injection sites include the lateral upper arm and thigh, abdomen, and upper back.

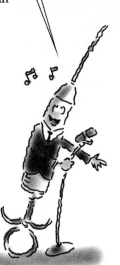

Now here's a song that'll take you back... "I've got you under my skin..."

- There are six steps to performing a subQ injection:

    Choose the injection site.

    Clean the skin.

    If the patient is thin, pinch the skin between your fingers and insert the needle at a 45-degree angle. If the patient is obese, insert the needle into the fatty tissue at a 90-degree angle.

    Aspirate for blood to make sure the needle isn't in a vein (unless injecting insulin or heparin).

    Administer the injection.

    Massage the site after removing the needle to enhance absorption; don't massage after giving heparin or insulin.

I.M. injections

- The drug is injected into a muscle.
- Common uses include:
    - administering drugs that need to be absorbed quickly
    - giving drugs in a large volume
    - preventing tissue irritation (can occur with shallow administration routes).

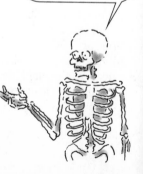

Honest... it isn't that I'm scared of needles. I just don't have a muscle to spare!

- A volume ranging from 0.5 to 3 ml may be given I.M.
  - A 3-ml injection may be given in the dorsogluteal, ventral gluteal, or vastus lateralis muscle.
  - Injections less than 3 ml may be given in the rectus femoris or deltoid muscle.
- Needles are 1″ to 3″ long and 18G to 23G.
- There are six steps to performing an I.M. injection:

  Choose the injection site.

  Clean the skin.

  Insert the needle at a 75- to 90-degree angle using a quick, dartlike action.

  Aspirate for blood to make sure the needle isn't in a vein.

  Push the plunger while holding the syringe steady.

  After injecting the drug, pull the needle straight out and apply pressure to the site.

Types of syringes

- Hypodermic syringes used for parenteral drugs come in three basic types:

   Standard syringes

   Tuberculin syringes

   Prefilled syringes.

Standard syringes

- Standard syringes are available in 3-, 5-, 10-, 20-, 40-, 50-, and 60-ml sizes.
- They all have a plunger, a barrel, a hub, a needle, and a dead space; the calibration marked on the syringe allows for accurate dose measurement.
- To administer a drug with a standard syringe, first check the "five rights" of medication administration and then follow these steps:
  - Use aseptic technique.
  - Calculate the dose.
  - Draw the drug into the syringe.
  - Pull the plunger back until the top ring of the plunger's black portion aligns with the correct calibration mark.
  - Double-check the dose measurement.
  - Administer the drug.

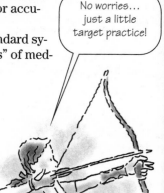

No worries... just a little target practice!

Anatomy of a syringe

Standard syringes come in many different sizes, but each syringe has the same components. This illustration shows the parts of a standard syringe.

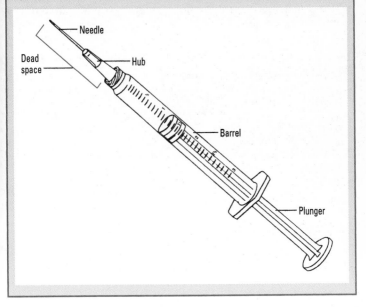

Tuberculin syringes

- Tuberculin syringes are commonly used for intradermal injections and to administer small amounts of drugs.
- Each syringe is calibrated to hundredths of a milliliter on the right and minims on the left.
- Measure drugs in a tuberculin syringe as you would in a standard syringe.

Touring a tuberculin syringe

A tuberculin syringe has the same components as a standard syringe. However, size and calibration of the syringe are distinct. Because the measurements on the tuberculin syringe are so small, take extra care when reading the dose.

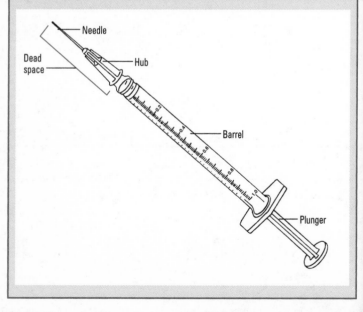

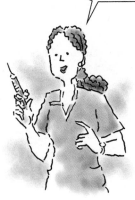

Remember, when you're using a tuberculin syringe for an intradermal injection, you're only giving a tiny amount of drug or serum. So check your measurements carefully.

Prefilled syringes

- These sterile syringes are packaged with a premeasured dose of a drug.
- They usually come with a cartridge-needle unit; some require use of a special holder, called a *Carpuject* or *Tubex*, to release the drug from the cartridge.
- Each cartridge is calibrated in tenths of a milliliter and has larger marks at half and full milliliter points.

Perusing a prefilled syringe

This illustration shows the parts of a prefilled syringe. Take note of the holder at right. The most commonly used brands of prefilled syringes are Carpuject and Tubex.

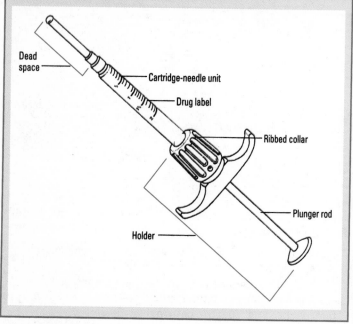

- In some cases, there's enough room in the cartridge to add a second drug (when a combined dose is ordered).
- Most manufacturers add a little extra drug in case some is lost when the air is purged.

- A special type of prefilled syringe, called a *closed-system device,* can be used to administer
  emergency drugs.
  - It has a needle and syringe in
    place and a separate prefilled
    drug chamber that must be
    connected to the syringe for
    use.
  - Atropine and lidocaine are ex-
    amples of drugs prepared this
    way.
- You can use the ratio-and-
  proportion method to calculate
  the dose of a drug available in a
  prefilled syringe.

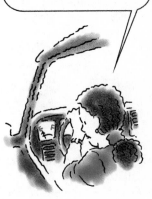

Rats... nearly empty!
Don't you wish all cars were
prefilled with an endless
supply of gas?

Learn by example

A prescriber orders *4 mg of I.M. morphine q3h* for your patient's pain. The drug is available in a prefilled syringe containing 10 mg of morphine/ml. How many milliliters of morphine
should you discard?

- Set up the first fraction using the known morphine concentration:

$$\frac{10 \text{ mg}}{1 \text{ ml}}$$

- Set up the second fraction with the desired dose and the unknown amount of morphine:

$$\frac{4 \text{ mg}}{X}$$

- Put these fractions into a proportion:

$$\frac{10 \text{ mg}}{1 \text{ ml}} = \frac{4 \text{ mg}}{X}$$

- Cross-multiply the fractions:

$$10 \text{ mg} \times X = 4 \text{ mg} \times 1 \text{ ml}$$

- Solve for X by dividing each side of the equation by 10 mg and canceling units that appear in both the numerator and denominator:

$$\frac{\cancel{10 \text{ mg}} \times X}{\cancel{10 \text{ mg}}} = \frac{4 \cancel{\text{ mg}} \times 1 \text{ ml}}{10 \cancel{\text{ mg}}}$$

$$X = \frac{4 \text{ ml}}{10}$$

$$X = 0.4 \text{ ml}$$

- The amount of morphine to give the patient is 0.4 ml. To calculate the amount to be discarded, subtract the ordered dose from the entire contents of the syringe:

$$
\begin{array}{rcl}
1.0 \text{ ml} & = & 10 \text{ mg morphine} \\
- \quad 0.4 \text{ ml} & = & 4 \text{ mg morphine} \\
\hline
0.6 \text{ ml} & = & 6 \text{ mg morphine}
\end{array}
$$

- The amount of morphine to discard is 0.6 ml.

> Calculating sample problems like this one keeps you on the cutting edge of clinical practice. Stay sharp!

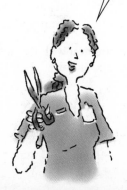

Types of needles

- Five different types of needles are used to inject parenteral drugs.

   Intradermal

   SubQ

   I.M.

   I.V.

  Filter

Choosing a needle

- When choosing a needle, consider the following:
  - Gauge—the inside diameter of the needle; the smaller the gauge, the larger the diameter.
  - Bevel—the angle at which the needle tip is opened; the bevel may be short, medium, or long.
  - Length—the distance from the needle tip to the needle hub; the length may vary from $3/8''$ to $3''$.

Choosing the right needle

When choosing a needle, consider its purpose as well as its gauge, bevel, and length. Use this selection guide to choose the right needles for your patients.

Intradermal needles
Intradermal needles are $^3/_8$" to $^5/_8$" long, usually have short bevels, and are 25G to 27G in diameter.

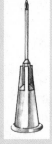

I.M. needles
I.M. needles are 1" to 3" long, have medium bevels, and are 18G to 23G in diameter.

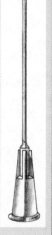

Subcutaneous needles
Subcutaneous needles are $^1/_2$" to $^5/_8$" long, have medium bevels, and are 23G to 28G in diameter.

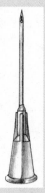

Choosing the right needle (continued)

I.V. needles

I.V. needles are 1" to 3" long, have long bevels, and are 14G to 25G in diameter.

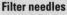

Filter needles

Filter needles are used for preparing a solution from a vial or ampule and shouldn't be used for injections. They're $1\frac{1}{2}$" long, have medium bevels, and are 20G in diameter.

Microscopic pieces of rubber or glass can enter the solution when you puncture the diaphragm of a vial with a needle or snap open an ampule. You can use a filter needle with a screening device in the hub to remove minute particles of foreign material from a solution.

Remember: After the medication is prepared, discard the filter needle!

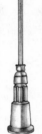

You don't need to go looking for a needle in a haystack—consider the needle's purpose, gauge, bevel, and length to narrow down your search.

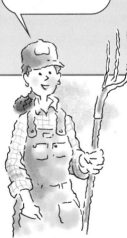

Interpreting drug labels

- You must read the label carefully to safely administer a parenteral drug.

Close up and label-able

This label shows the information you need to know to safely administer a parenteral drug.

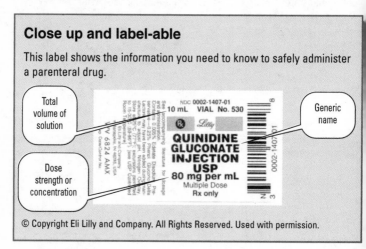

- Parenteral drugs are packaged in glass ampules, in single- or multiple-dose vials with rubber stoppers, and in prefilled syringes and cartridges; the packaging should clearly state that the drugs are used for injection.
- Reading the label is similar to reading the label of an oral drug; check for:
  - trade name
  - generic name
  - total volume of solution in the container
  - dose strength or concentration
  - approved routes of administration
  - expiration date
  - special instructions, as needed.

Solution components

- A *solute* is the liquid or solid form of a drug.
- A *solution* is a liquid that contains a solute dissolved in a diluent or solvent.
- Normal saline solution is a solution of salt (the solute) in purified water (the solvent).

> Here's a tricky problem... how to fit a large amount of drug into a small glass of water. Sure hope the solution presents itself soon!

Interpreting percentage solutions

You can determine the contents of a weight per volume (W/V) or volume per volume (V/V) percentage solution by reading the label, as shown here.

What the label says	What the solution contains
0.9% (W/V) NaCl	0.9 g of sodium chloride in 100 ml of finished solution
5% (W/V) boric acid solution	5 g of boric acid in 100 ml of finished solution
5% (W/V) dextrose	5 g of dextrose in 100 ml of finished solution
2% (V/V) hydrogen peroxide	2 ml of hydrogen peroxide in 100 ml of finished solution
70% (V/V) isopropyl alcohol	70 ml of isopropyl alcohol in 100 ml of finished solution
10% (V/V) glycerin	10 ml of glycerin in 100 ml of finished solution

Solution strengths

- Solutions come in different strengths, which are expressed on the drug label as percentage solutions or ratio solutions.
- A clear way to label or describe a solution is as a percentage.
- On the label, the solution may be expressed as weight per volume (W/V) or volume per volume (V/V).
  - In a W/V solution, the percentage or strength refers to the number of grams of solute per 100 ml of reconstituted solution.
  - In a V/V solution, the percentage refers to the number of milliliters of solute per 100 ml of finished solution.
  - Mathematically, these would be expressed as follows:

$$\% = \frac{\text{weight}}{\text{volume}} = \frac{\text{grams solute}}{100 \text{ ml finished solution}}$$

$$\% = \frac{\text{volume}}{\text{volume}} = \frac{\text{milliliters solute}}{100 \text{ ml finished solution}}$$

- A solution may also be described as a ratio.

Interpreting ratio solutions

You can determine the contents of a weight per volume (W : V) or volume per volume (V : V) ratio solution from the label, as shown here.

What the label reads	What the solution contains
benzalkonium chloride 1 : 750 (W : V)	1 g of benzalkonium chloride in 750 ml of finished solution
silver nitrate 1 : 100 (W : V)	1 g of silver nitrate in 100 ml of finished solution
hydrogen peroxide 2 : 100 (V : V)	2 ml of hydrogen peroxide in 100 ml of finished solution
glycerin 10 : 100 (V : V)	10 ml of glycerin in 100 ml of finished solution

- The strength of a ratio solution is expressed as two numbers separated by a colon.
  - In a weight per volume (W : V) solution, the first number signifies the amount of a drug in grams.
  - In a volume per volume (V : V) solution, the first number signifies the amount of drug in milliliters; the second signifies the volume of finished solution in milliliters.
  - This may be expressed as follows:

  Ratio = amount of drug : amount of finished solution.

Insulin and unit-based drugs

- Insulin, heparin, and penicillin G are parenteral drugs that are measured in units.
- The number of units appears on the drug label.

Look for the unit label

The label of a parenteral drug that's measured in units includes the information shown here.

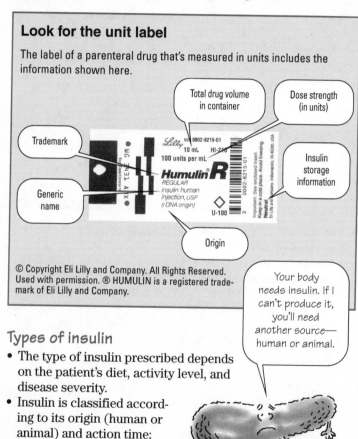

Total drug volume in container

Dose strength (in units)

Trademark

Insulin storage information

Generic name

Origin

© Copyright Eli Lilly and Company. All Rights Reserved. Used with permission. ® HUMULIN is a registered trademark of Eli Lilly and Company.

Your body needs insulin. If I can't produce it, you'll need another source— human or animal.

Types of insulin

- The type of insulin prescribed depends on the patient's diet, activity level, and disease severity.
- Insulin is classified according to its origin (human or animal) and action time; origin appears on the drug label.

- Most insulin labels also contain an initial after the trade name, indicating the type of insulin, which varies according to onset, peak, and duration of action:
  – R for regular insulin
  – L for lente insulin

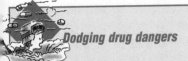

Dodging drug dangers

Identifying insulin subtypes

Insulin labels must be read carefully because they may contain confusingly similar information. Remember that one type of insulin, such as lente, may come in different subtypes, but those subtypes aren't interchangeable. For example, if the prescriber orders lente human insulin zinc suspension, don't substitute lente purified pork insulin zinc suspension USP. Otherwise, a hypersensitive patient could develop a severe allergic reaction.

Type	Subtype
Lente	• Lente human insulin zinc suspension (semisynthetic) • Lente purified pork insulin zinc suspension USP
NPH	• NPH human insulin isophane suspension USP • NPH purified pork insulin isophane suspension USP • 70% NPH, human insulin isophane suspension and 30% regular, human insulin injection (semisynthetic)
Regular	• Regular human insulin injection (semisynthetic) USP • Regular insulin, insulin injection USP (pork) • Regular purified pork insulin injection USP
Ultralente	• Ultralente insulin, extended insulin zinc suspension USP • Ultralente human extended insulin zinc suspension

  – U for ultralente insulin
  – N for neutral protamine Hagedorn (NPH).
- Insulin doses are available in two concentrations:
  – U-100 insulin, which contains 100 units of insulin per milliliter (the most common concentration)
  – U-500 insulin, which contains 500 units/ml (given to patients requiring large doses of insulin).

Insulin syringes

- The U-100 syringe is the only type available in the United States.
- It's calibrated so that 1 ml holds 100 units of insulin.
- A low-dose U-100 syringe may hold 30 or 50 units of insulin or less.

Selecting an insulin syringe

These syringes are examples of the different dose-specific insulin syringes that are available. The 1-ml U-100 syringe delivers up to 100 units of insulin. The low-dose $3/10$-ml and $1/2$-ml syringes deliver up to 30 or 50 units of U-100 insulin.

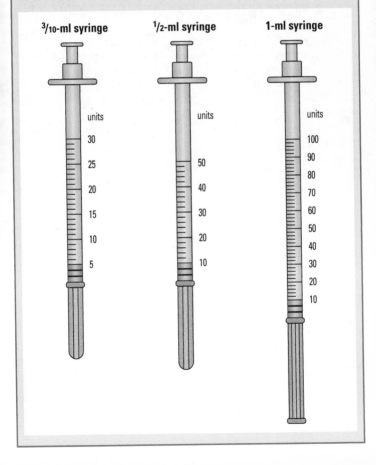

Reading insulin orders

- Insulin orders are based on the patient's blood glucose readings.
- It may take several dosage adjustments to get an accurate dose.

Insulin action times

Insulin preparations are modified through combination with larger insoluble protein molecules to slow absorption and prolong activity. An insulin preparation may be rapid-acting, intermediate-acting, or long-acting, as shown in this table.

Drug	Onset	Peak	Duration
Rapid-acting			
regular insulin	$1/2$ to 1 hr	2 to 3 hr	6 to 12 hr
lispro insulin	$< 1/4$ hr	$1/2$ to $1 1/2$ hr	6 to 8 hr
Intermediate-acting			
insulin zinc suspension (lente)	1 to $2 1/2$ hr	7 to 15 hr	24 hr
isophane insulin suspension (NPH)	1 to $1 1/2$ hr	4 to 12 hr	24 hr
isophane 70%, regular insulin 30%	$1/2$ hr	2 to 12 hr	24 hr
isophane 50%, regular insulin 50%	$1/2$ hr	4 to 8 hr	24 hr
Long-acting			
extended insulin zinc suspension (ultralente)	4 to 8 hr	10 to 30 hr	> 36 hr
insulin glargine (Lantus)	1 hr	5 hr	24 hr

- In the inpatient setting, the prescriber may write a sliding-scale order; this individualizes the patient's insulin doses and administration times according to several variables, including:
  - age
  - activity level
  - desired degree of blood glucose control
  - response to insulin.
- An order for a patient receiving regular insulin on a sliding scale might appear as follows:

Start regular insulin sliding scale:

Blood glucose value	Insulin dose
Less than 180 mg/dl	No insulin
180 to 240 mg/dl	10 units regular insulin subQ
241 to 400 mg/dl	20 units regular insulin subQ
> 400 mg/dl	Call prescriber for orders

- Always administer U-100 insulin unless the order specifies U-500 insulin.

> A sliding scale allows you to individualize the patient's insulin doses until you can get a handle on his actual dosage needs. Now if I can just get a handle on these new skates...

Combining insulins

- An order may be written to combine two insulins.
- If the insulins are regular and NPH, they can be combined into the same syringe following this procedure:
  - Read the insulin order carefully.
  - Read the vial labels carefully, noting the type, concentration, source, and expiration date of the drugs.
  - Roll the NPH vial between your palms to mix it thoroughly.
  - Choose the appropriate syringes.
  - Clean the tops of both vials of insulin with alcohol swabs.
  - Inject air into the NPH vial equal to the amount of insulin you need to give.
  - Withdraw the needle and syringe, but don't withdraw any NPH insulin.
  - Inject an amount of air equal to the dose of the regular insulin into the regular insulin vial. Then invert or tilt the vial and withdraw the prescribed amount of regular insulin into the syringe. Draw the clear, regular insulin first to avoid contamination by the cloudy, longer-acting insulin.

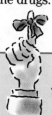

Memory jogger

If you have trouble remembering which insulin to draw first, think of the phrase "clear before cloudy." (Who doesn't prefer a clear day to a cloudy day?)

This phrase also reminds you how these drugs work: A clear day seems short, but a cloudy day seems to go on forever. Clear regular insulin is short-acting and cloudy NPH insulin is long-acting.

- Clean the top of the NPH vial again. Then insert the needle of the syringe containing the regular insulin into the vial, and withdraw the prescribed amount of NPH insulin.
- Mix the insulins in the syringe by pulling back slightly on the plunger and tilting the syringe back and forth.
- Recheck the drug order.
- Have a second nurse verify the withdrawn dose and cosign the medication administration record.
- Administer the insulin immediately.

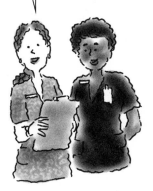

Always read insulin orders carefully, and follow all procedures when combining drugs, including having another nurse verify the dose and cosign the medication record.

Learn by example

The prescriber writes an order for a patient to receive *7,000 units of heparin subQ q12h.* The heparin you have available contains 10,000 units/ml. How many milliliters of heparin should you give?

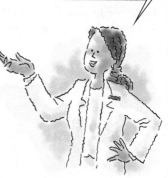

This calculation concerns heparin—another unit-based parenteral drug.

• Set up the first ratio with the known heparin concentration:

10,000 ml : 1 ml

• Set up the second ratio with the desired dose and the unknown amount of heparin:

7,000 units : X

• Put these ratios into a proportion:

10,000 units : 1 ml :: 7,000 units : X

• Set up an equation by multiplying the means and extremes:

1 ml × 7,000 units = 10,000 units × X

• Solve for X by dividing each side of the equation by 10,000 units and canceling units that appear in both the numerator and denominator:

$$\frac{1\,ml \times 7,000\ \cancel{units}}{10,000\ \cancel{units}} = \frac{10,000\ \cancel{units} \times X}{10,000\ \cancel{units}}$$

$$X = 0.7\ ml$$

• You should give the patient 0.7 ml of heparin.

Reconstituting powders

- Drugs that become unstable in solution are packaged as powders.
- Powders come in single-strength or multiple-strength formulations.
  - Single-strength powders can only be reconstituted to one dose strength per administration route.
  - A multiple-strength powder can be reconstituted to various dose strengths by adjusting the amount of diluent.
  - When reconstituting a multiple-strength powder, check the drug label or package insert for the dose-strength options and choose the one that's closest to the ordered strength.

How to reconstitute

- Begin by checking the label of the powder container.
- The label will tell you:
  - the quantity of the drug in a vial or ampule
  - the amount and type of diluent to add to the powder
  - the strength and expiration date of the resulting solution.
- Keep in mind that, when diluent is added to a powder, the fluid volume increases. That's why the label calls for less diluent than the total volume of prepared solution.

- Also be aware that some drugs come in a vial with two chambers that are separated by a rubber stopper.
- Add the appropriate amount of diluent to the powder.

Two chambers (one's a powder room!)

Some drugs that require reconstitution are packaged in vials with two chambers separated by a rubber stopper. In the illustration below, note that the upper chamber contains the diluent and the lower chamber contains the powder. The plunger is depressed to inject the diluent into the powder.

> There's no real trick to adding a diluent. Just read the powder's label, and select the right type and amount.

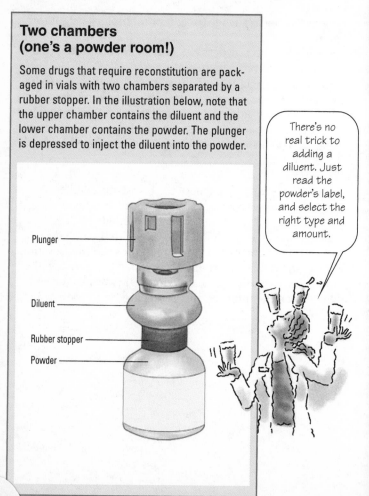

Plunger

Diluent

Rubber stopper

Powder

After you reconstitute

- Check the label or package insert for special instructions about administration and storage after reconstitution.
- After reconstituting the drug, label it with your initials, the reconstitution date, expiration date, and dose strength.

Ready to administer

- To determine how much reconstituted drug you need to give your patient, refer to the drug label for information about the dose strength of the prepared solution.
- For example, to give 500 mg of a drug when the dose strength of the solution is 1 g (or 1,000 mg)/10 ml, set up a proportion with fractions as follows:

$$\frac{X}{500 \text{ mg}} = \frac{10 \text{ ml}}{1,000 \text{ mg}}$$

- Cross-multiply the fractions:

$$X \times 1,000 \text{ mg} = 500 \text{ mg} \times 10 \text{ ml}$$

- Solve for X by dividing both sides of the equation by 1,000 mg and canceling units that appear in the numerator and denominator:

$$\frac{X \times \cancel{1,000 \text{ mg}}}{\cancel{1,000 \text{ mg}}} = \frac{500 \cancel{\text{ mg}} \times 10 \text{ ml}}{1,000 \cancel{\text{ mg}}}$$

$$X = \frac{5,000 \text{ ml}}{1,000}$$

$$X = 5 \text{ ml}$$

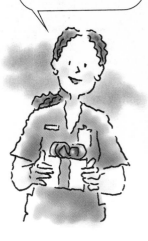

Sometimes, when the information isn't clearly labeled on the outside, you need to think—and look—inside the box.

- If the dose-strength information isn't on the drug label, check the package insert.

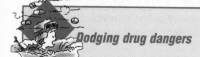

Dodging drug dangers

Inspect the insert

The package inserts that are included with drugs commonly provide a great deal of information that may not be on the outer label. For example, the drug label for ceftazidime provides no information about reconstitution, but the package insert does. These are the possible diluent combinations as they appear in the package insert that comes with this drug.

Vial size	Diluent to be added	Approximate ml available	Approximate average concentration
I.M. or I.V. direct (bolus) injection			
1 g	3 ml	3.6 ml	280 mg/ml
I.V. infusion			
1 g	10 ml	10.6 ml	95 mg/ml
2 g	10 ml	11.2 ml	180 mg/ml

Learn by example

Your patient has an order to receive 100,000 units of penicillin, but the only available vial holds 1 million units. The drug label says to add 4.5 ml of normal saline solution to yield 1 million units/5 ml. How much solution should you administer after reconstituting?

- First, dilute the powder according to the instructions on the label. Then set up the first fraction with the known penicillin concentration:

$$\frac{1,000,000 \text{ units}}{5 \text{ ml}}$$

- Set up the second fraction with the desired dose and the unknown amount of solution:

$$\frac{100,000 \text{ units}}{X}$$

- Put these fractions into a proportion:

$$\frac{1,000,000 \text{ units}}{5 \text{ ml}} = \frac{100,000 \text{ units}}{X}$$

- Cross-multiply the fractions:

$$5 \text{ ml} \times 100,000 \text{ units} = X \times 1,000,000 \text{ units}$$

- Solve for X by dividing each side of the equation by 1 million units and canceling units that appear in both the numerator and denominator:

$$\frac{5\ ml \times 100{,}000\ \text{units}}{1{,}000{,}000\ \text{units}} = \frac{X \times 1{,}000{,}000\ \text{units}}{1{,}000{,}000\ \text{units}}$$

$$X = \frac{5{,}000{,}000\ ml}{1{,}000{,}000}$$

$$X = 0.5\ ml$$

- The amount of solution that yields 100,000 units of penicillin after reconstitution is 0.5 ml.

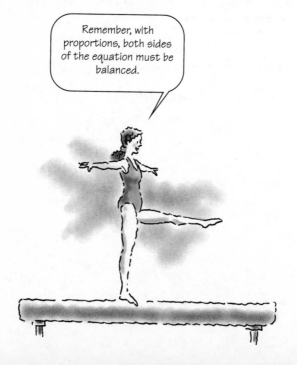

Remember, with proportions, both sides of the equation must be balanced.

I.V. infusions

6

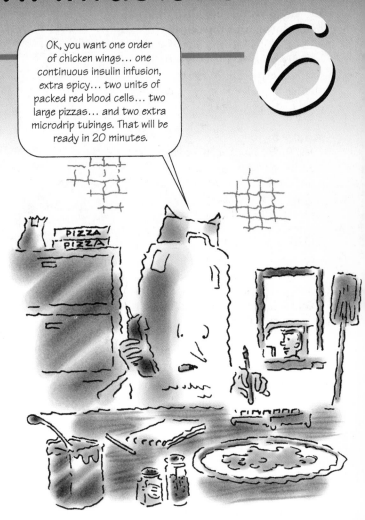

Preparing and administering I.V. infusions

- I.V. therapy—the administration of liquid substances directly into a vein—is typically the quickest way to deliver medications and fluids to the body; certain substances, such as blood, can only be delivered by the I.V. route.

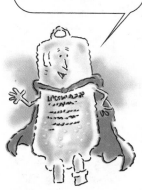

> That's right... I'm known for my speedy— sometimes lifesaving— delivery of medications and fluids.

- Some commonly infused substances include:
  - I.V. fluids (such as normal saline or dextrose solutions)
  - analgesics
  - heparin and insulin
  - electrolyte and nutrition solutions
  - blood and blood products
  - total parenteral nutrition (TPN).
- Rapid infusion of I.V. fluids or blood products could seriously threaten the patient's health.
- To administer I.V. fluids safely, you need to know:
  - how much fluid to give
  - length of time to administer the fluid
  - type of fluid to give
  - what needs to be added to the fluid.
- You should be able to identify all the components of an I.V. fluid by examining the outside of the I.V. bag.

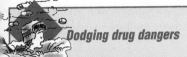

Dodging drug dangers

Read the bag

The outside of an I.V. bag is an important source of information for calculating infusion rates and times. Read it carefully!

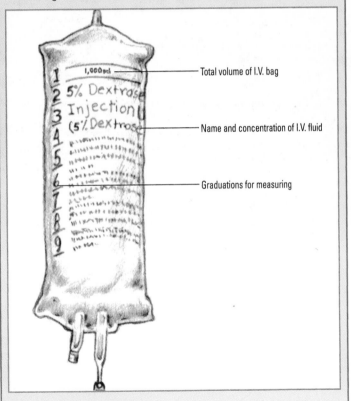

- You need to be able to select the proper tubing, calculate the drip rate and flow rate, and be comfortable with I.V. infusion equipment and procedures.

Help desk

Checking an I.V.

You can save time by assessing your patient's I.V. infusion at the beginning of every shift.

Performing checks early helps avoid confusion when your shift gets busy.

- Are the time, volume, and rate labeled correctly? If so, do they match the order?
- Check maintenance fluids and drug infusions, such as insulin, dopamine, and morphine. Are the additives correct? Are they in the right solutions?
- After calculating the drug dosage, check the bag again to verify that the solution is labeled with the time, name, and amount of drug added.
- If an electronic infusion device is being used, is it set correctly?
- Examine the tubing from the bag down to the patient to see whether the drug is infusing into the correct I.V. port. This is critical when a patient has multiple lines.

Selecting appropriate tubing

- I.V. tubing comes in two sizes: micro-drip and macrodrip
  - Microdrip tubing delivers smaller drops, allowing more drops to flow per minute; it's more appropriate for a slower infusion rate.
  - Macrodrip tubing delivers larger drops, allowing fewer drops to flow per minute; it's more appropriate for a faster infusion rate.
- After selecting the tubing, determine the drip rate.

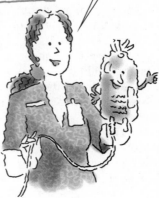

Remember to choose your tubing wisely!

Help desk

Tube tips

Follow these rules when selecting I.V. tubing:
- Use macrodrip tubing for infusions of at least 80 ml/hour.
- Use microdrip tubing for infusions of less than 80 ml/hour and for pediatric patients (to prevent fluid overload).
- With electronic infusion devices, select the tubing specifically made to work with those devices.

Calculating the drip rate

- The *drip rate* is the number of drops of solution you want to infuse per minute.
- To calculate the drip rate, you first need to know the calibration of the I.V. tubing selected.
- The *drop factor* is the number of drops per milliliter of solution calibrated for an administration set; it's listed on the I.V. tubing package.
  - Standard (macrodrip) tubing usually has a drop factor of 10, 15, or 20 gtt/ml.
  - Microdrip tubing is usually 60 gtt/ml.
- To calculate the drip rate, use this formula:

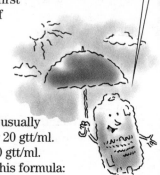

With all this talk about drip rates and drop factors, I suspect we're in for a little rain. Glad I have my umbrella handy!

$$\text{Drip rate in drops/minute} = \frac{\text{Total milliliters}}{\text{Total minutes}} \times \frac{\text{Drop factor}}{\text{in drops/ml}}$$

Learn by example

Your patient needs an infusion of dextrose 5% in water (D_5W) at 125 ml/hour. If the tubing set is calibrated at 15 gtt/ml, what's the drip rate?

- First, convert 1 hour to 60 minutes to fit the formula.
- Then set up a fraction. Place the volume of the infusion in the numerator. Place the number of minutes in which the volume is to be infused in the denominator:

$$\frac{125 \text{ ml}}{60 \text{ minutes}}$$

- To determine X—or the number of drops per minute to be infused—multiply the fraction by the drop factor. Cancel units that appear in both the numerator and denominator:

$$X = \frac{125 \text{ ~~ml~~}}{60 \text{ minutes}} \times \frac{15 \text{ gtt}}{\text{~~ml~~}}$$

- Solve for X by dividing the numerator by the denominator:

$$X = \frac{125 \times 15 \text{ gtt}}{60 \text{ minutes}}$$

$$X = \frac{1,875 \text{ gtt}}{60 \text{ minutes}}$$

$$X = 31.25$$

- The drip rate is 31.25 gtt/minute, rounded to 31 gtt/minute.

Calculating the flow rate

- If the patient is receiving a large-volume infusion to maintain hydration or to replace fluids or electrolytes, you may need to know the flow rate.
- The flow rate is the number of milliliters of fluid to administer over 1 hour.
- To determine the flow rate, use this formula:

$$\text{Flow rate} = \frac{\text{Total volume ordered}}{\text{Number of hours}}$$

Learn by example

Your patient needs 1,000 ml of fluid over 8 hours.

- Find the flow rate by dividing the volume by the number of hours:

$$\text{Flow rate} = \frac{1{,}000 \text{ ml}}{8 \text{ hours}} = 125 \text{ ml/hour}$$

- The flow rate is 125 ml/hour.

Quick calculation of drip rates (based on flow rate)

- There's a shortcut for calculating I.V. drip rates that's based on the fact that all drop factors can be evenly divided into 60 (the number of minutes in 1 hour).
- For macrodrip sets, use these rules:
  - For sets that deliver 10 gtt/ml, divide the hourly flow rate by 6.
  - For sets that deliver 15 gtt/ml, divide the hourly flow rate by 4.
  - For sets that deliver 20 gtt/ml, divide the hourly flow rate by 3.
- With a microdrip set, simply remember that the drip rate is the same as the flow rate.

> Anything that saves me a little time—like these rules for quick calculation of drip rates—is well worth the reading. Don't you agree?

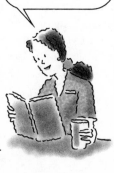

Learn by example

The prescriber orders 1,000 ml of normal saline solution to be infused over 12 hours. If your administration set delivers 15 gtt/ml, what's the drip rate?

- First, determine the flow rate *(X)* by dividing the number of milliliters to be delivered by the number of hours:

$$X = \frac{1{,}000 \text{ ml}}{12 \text{ hours}} = 83.3 \text{ ml/hour}$$

- Remember the rule: for sets that deliver 15 gtt/ml, divide the flow rate by 4 to determine the drip rate:

$$X = \frac{83.3}{4}$$

$$X = 20.8$$

- The drip rate is 20.8 gtt/minute, rounded to 21 gtt/minute.

Calculating the infusion time

- After calculating the flow rate and drip rate, compute the *infusion time*—the time required to infuse a specified volume of fluid.
- Knowing the infusion time will help keep the infusion on schedule and determine when to start the next infusion.
- To calculate the infusion time, use this formula:

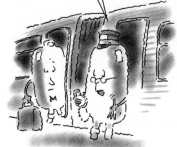

All aboard! We've got a schedule to keep!

$$\text{Infusion time} = \frac{\text{Volume to be infused}}{\text{Flow rate}}$$

- Alternatively, if you know the volume to be infused as well as the drip rate and drop factor, use this formula to calculate the infusion time:

$$\text{infusion time in hours} = \frac{\text{volume to be infused}}{(\text{drip rate} \div \text{drop factor}) \times 60 \text{ minutes}}$$

Learn by example

If you plan to infuse 1 L of D_5W at 50 ml/hour, what's the infusion time?

- First, convert 1 L to 1,000 ml to make equivalent units of measurement.
- Then set up the fraction with the volume of the infusion as the numerator and the flow rate as the denominator:

$$\frac{1,000 \text{ ml}}{50 \text{ ml/hour}}$$

- Next, solve for X by dividing 1,000 by 50 and canceling units that appear in both the numerator and denominator:

$$X = \frac{1,000 \text{ m\mkern-11mu/\mkern-3mul}}{50 \text{ m\mkern-11mu/\mkern-3mul/hour}}$$

$$X = 20 \text{ hours}$$

- The D_5W will infuse in 20 hours.

Learn by example

A prescriber orders 250 ml of normal saline solution I.V. at 32 gtt/minute. The drop factor is 15 gtt/ml. What's the infusion time?

- First, set up the formula with the information you know:

$$\text{infusion time} \atop \text{in hours} = \frac{250 \text{ ml}}{(32 \text{ gtt/minute} \div 15 \text{ gtt/ml}) \times 60 \text{ minutes}}$$

- Then divide the drip rate by the drop factor. (Remember: To divide a complex fraction, multiply the dividend by the reciprocal of the divisor.)
- Cancel units that appear in both the numerator and denominator.

$$\frac{32 \text{ g\mkern-13mu/\mkern-3mutt}}{1 \text{ min}} \times \frac{1 \text{ ml}}{15 \text{ g\mkern-13mu/\mkern-3mutt}} = \frac{32 \text{ ml}}{15 \text{ min}} = 2.13 \text{ ml/minute}$$

Now, rewrite the equation (solve for X) with the result placed in the denominator. Cancel units that appear in both the numerator and denominator:

$$X = \frac{250 \; \cancel{ml}}{\dfrac{2.13 \; \cancel{ml}}{1 \; \cancel{min}} \times \dfrac{60 \; \cancel{min}}{1 \; hour}}$$

To find the infusion time, solve for X:

$$X = \frac{250}{2.13 \times 60 \; hours}$$

$$X = \frac{250}{127.8 \; hours}$$

Round off the denominator and then divide it into the numerator:

$$X = \frac{250}{128 \; hours}$$

$$X = 1.95 \; hours$$

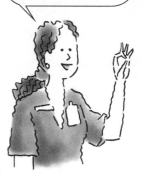

When working with infusion times, it's OK to round off hours. However, remember to convert the decimal fraction portion of time to minutes.

The infusion time is 1.95 hours. Convert the decimal fraction portion of time to minutes by multiplying by 60:

$$0.95 \; hour \times 60 \; minutes = 57 \; minutes$$

The infusion time is 1 hour and 57 minutes.

Regulating infusions

- Infusions can be regulated manually or with a pump.
- Patient-controlled analgesia (PCA) pumps allow the patient to self-administer an analgesic.

Manual regulation

- To manually regulate the I.V. flow rate, count the number of drops going into the drip chamber.
- While counting the drops, adjust the flow with the roller clamp until the fluid is infusing at the appropriate number of drops per minute.

> Save time. Calculate the drip rate for 15 seconds instead of a minute. Divide the prescribed rate by four.

- Calculate the drip rate for 15 seconds only, and then divide the prescribed drip rate by 4 because 15 seconds is $\frac{1}{4}$ of a minute.
- After achieving the correct drip rate, time-tape the I.V. bag to ensure that the solution is given at the prescribed rate.

Electronic infusion pumps

- Electronic pumps administer fluid under positive pressure; they're calibrated by drip rate and volume to deliver a constant amount of solution per hour.
- Infusion pumps offer many advantages over standard (gravity-drip) devices:
  - easier control of the drip rate or volume, which can be set on the machine
  - less time needed to calculate an infusion rate
  - greater accuracy
  - less maintenance.

Help desk

Taped up and ready to drip

Time-taping an I.V. bag helps ensure that an I.V. solution is administered at the prescribed rate. It also helps facilitate recording of fluid intake.

To time-tape an I.V. bag, place a strip of adhesive tape from the top to the bottom of the bag, next to the fluid level markings. (This illustration shows a bag time-taped for a rate of 100 ml/hour beginning at 10 a.m.)

0 marks the spot

Next to the "0" marking, record the time that you hung the bag. Then knowing the hourly rate, mark each hour on the tape next to the corresponding fluid marking. At the bottom of the tape, mark the time at which the solution will be completely infused.

Ink alert

Don't write directly on the bag with a felt tip marker because the ink may seep into the fluid. Some manufacturers provide printed time-tapes for use with their solutions.

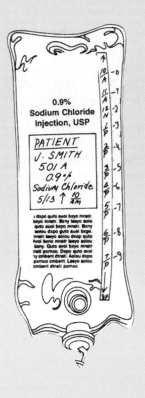

0.9%
Sodium Chloride
Injection, USP

PATIENT
J. SMITH
501 A
0.9 %
Sodium Chloride
5/13 ↑ 10 AM

- Most pumps keep track of the amount of fluid that's been infused.
- Many pumps have an alarm that signals when the fluid container is empty or when a mechanical problem occurs.
- Some pumps have variable pressure limits that prevent them from pumping fluid into an infiltrated or occluded site.

Regulating I.V. flow with a pump

- Program the infusion pump based on your calculation of the infusion rate.
- Always double-check the pump and count the drips in the chamber just as you would with manual regulation.
- To determine the pump settings, consider the volume of fluid to be given and the total infusion time. With most devices, you'll need to program the amount of fluid to be infused and the hourly flow rate.

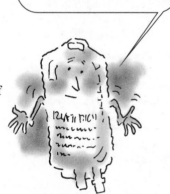

Given all the advantages and special features, it seems like an electronic pump would be the logical choice.

Patient-controlled analgesia pumps

- PCA pumps allow the patient to self-administer an analgesic by pushing a button.
- They're programmed to deliver a precise dose every time.
- They can also be programmed to deliver a basal dose of the drug in addition to the patient-controlled dose.

- The main advantages of using a PCA pump are:
  - the blood concentrations of analgesics remain consistent throughout the day
  - the patient tends to use less medication and feels a greater sense of control over his pain.
- PCA pumps have several safety features:
  - Drug dose and frequency of administration are programmed, preventing the patient from overmedicating himself.
  - An access code or key is required before entering the drug dose and frequency information; this prevents unauthorized users from resetting the pump.
  - Some PCA pumps record the number of patient requests and the number of times the patient receives the drug; this helps track the need for possible dosage adjustments.

PCA guidelines

- Follow these guidelines when preparing a PCA pump for a patient:
  - Draw the correct amount and concentration of the drug and insert it into the PCA pump. Most facilities use prefilled cartridges.

Using a PCA pump gives your patient the sense that he's in the driver's seat—or at least the co-pilot's seat—when it comes to his pain management.

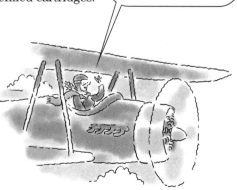

- – Program the pump according to the manufacturer's directions.
- – Carefully read the PCA log, and then record the information based on your facility's policy.
- When interpreting the PCA log, note several factors:
  - – Note the strength (number of milligrams per milliliter) of drug solution in the syringe.
  - – Note the number of times the patient received the drug throughout the time covered by your assessment (usually 4 hours).
  - – Multiply the number of injections by the volume of each injection and add the basal rate to determine the amount of solution the patient received.
  - – Multiply this amount by the solution strength to find the total amount of drug, using this formula:

  Fluid volume $\times$ Solution strength = Total drug received

- Record this amount in milligrams in the patient's medication administration record.

Adjusting the infusion rate

- If an adjustment needs to be made to the flow rate because the infusion is running too fast or too slow, recalculate the drip rate taking into account the remaining time and volume.

  - If the volume has infused too slowly, determine if the patient can tolerate an increased rate by assessing his cardiac and respiratory status.

  - If the volume has infused too quickly, slow or stop the infusion and assess the patient for signs of fluid overload. Call the practitioner if the patient has increased blood pressure or crackles.

Give me a second, and I'll be right over to help you with those adjustments.

- The infusion rate may need to be increased to perform a *fluid challenge*, which monitors how the patient tolerates increased fluid.
  - The fastest way to do a fluid challenge is by increasing the I.V. flow rate for a specified time and then reducing it to a maintenance rate.
  - Use extra caution when administering a fluid bolus to pediatric and elderly patients.

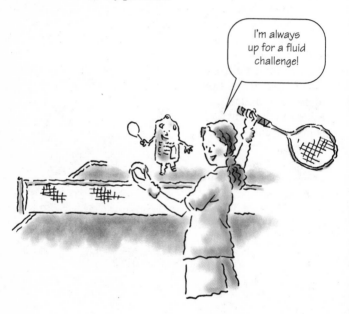

I'm always up for a fluid challenge!

Heparin and insulin infusions

- You may need to administer heparin or insulin as part of a large-volume I.V. infusion; both drugs are typically ordered in milliliters per hour or units per hour.
- Calculate the drug dose so that it falls within therapeutic limits. (See chapter 5, Parenteral drugs, for more information on heparin and insulin.)

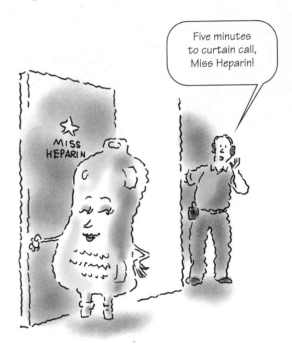

Calculating heparin infusions

- Heparin is ordered in doses of units per hour or milliliters per hour.
- Each dose is individualized based on the patient's coagulation status as measured by the partial thromboplastin time (PTT).
- To calculate the hourly heparin flow rate, first determine the solution's concentration by dividing the units of drug added to the bag by the number of milliliters of solution. Then write a fraction stating the desired dose of heparin over the unknown flow rate.

> When it comes to heparin infusions, keep it individual... measure your patient's PTT and treat him like a VIP!

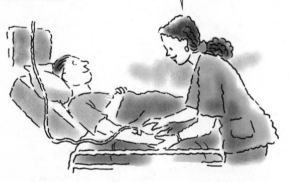

- If a heparin infusion is ordered in milliliters per hour, you should calculate it in units per hour to make sure that the dose falls within a therapeutic range.

Learn by example

An order states *heparin 40,000 units in 1 L of D_5W I.V. Infuse at 1,000 units/hour*. What's the flow rate in milliliters per hour?

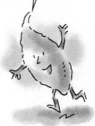

Sorry... can't stop to chat until you solve for X and figure out the precise flow rate for this patient!

- First, convert 1 L to 1,000 ml. Then write a fraction to express the known solution strength:

$$\frac{40,000 \text{ units}}{1,000 \text{ ml}}$$

- Write a second fraction with the desired dose of heparin in the numerator and the unknown flow rate in the denominator:

$$\frac{1,000 \text{ units/hour}}{X}$$

- Put these fractions into a proportion:

$$\frac{40,000 \text{ units}}{1,000 \text{ ml}} = \frac{1,000 \text{ units/hour}}{X}$$

- To find the flow rate, solve for X by cross-multiplying:

$$40,000 \text{ units} \times X = 1,000 \text{ units/hour} \times 1,000 \text{ ml}$$

- Divide each side of the equation by 40,000 units and cancel units that appear in both the numerator and denominator:

$$\frac{\cancel{40,000\ units} \times X}{\cancel{40,000\ units}} = \frac{1,000\ \cancel{units}/hour \times 1,000\ ml}{40,000\ \cancel{units}}$$

$$X = \frac{1,000,000\ ml/hour}{40,000}$$

$$X = 25\ ml/hour$$

- To administer heparin at 1,000 units/hour, you should set the flow rate at 25 ml/hour.

Learn by example

A patient is receiving 20,000 units of heparin in 1,000 ml of D_5W I.V. at a rate of 30 ml/hour. What heparin dose is the patient receiving?

- Write a fraction to describe the known solution strength:

$$\frac{20,000\ units}{1,000\ ml}$$

- Set up a second fraction with the flow rate in the denominator and the unknown dose of heparin in the numerator:

$$\frac{X}{30\ ml/hour}$$

- Put these fractions into a proportion:

$$\frac{20,000\ units}{1,000\ ml} = \frac{X}{30\ ml/hour}$$

- Solve for X by cross-multiplying:

$$1,000\ ml \times X = 30\ ml/hour \times 20,000\ units$$

- Divide each side of the equation by 1,000 ml, and cancel units that appear in both the numerator and denominator:

$$\frac{\cancel{1,000 \text{ ml}} \times X}{\cancel{1,000 \text{ ml}}} = \frac{30 \text{ } \cancel{\text{ml}}\text{/hour} \times 20,000 \text{ units}}{1,000 \text{ } \cancel{\text{ml}}}$$

$$X = \frac{30 \times 20,000 \text{ units/hour}}{1,000}$$

$$X = \frac{600,000 \text{ units/hour}}{1,000}$$

$$X = 600 \text{ units/hour}$$

- With the flow rate set at 30 ml/hour, the patient is receiving a heparin dose of 600 units/hour.

Calculating continuous insulin infusions

- A continuous insulin infusion allows close control of insulin administration based on serial measurements of blood glucose levels.
- It must be administered with an infusion pump.
- Insulin is usually prescribed in units per hour, but it may be ordered in milliliters per hour.
- The infusion should be in a concentration of 1 unit/ml to avoid calculation errors.

Sorry... no time for siestas with continuous insulin infusions!

Learn by example

Your patient needs a continuous infusion of 150 units of regular insulin in 150 ml of normal saline solution at 6 units/hour. What's the flow rate?

- Write a fraction to describe the known solution strength:

$$\frac{150 \text{ units}}{150 \text{ ml}}$$

- Write a second fraction with the infusion rate in the numerator and the unknown flow rate in the denominator:

$$\frac{6 \text{ units/hour}}{X}$$

- Write the two fractions as a proportion:

$$\frac{150 \text{ units}}{150 \text{ ml}} = \frac{6 \text{ units/hour}}{X}$$

- Solve for X by cross-multiplying:

$$150 \text{ units} \times X = 6 \text{ units/hour} \times 150 \text{ ml}$$

- Divide each side of the equation by 150 units, and cancel units that appear in both the numerator and denominator:

$$\frac{\cancel{150 \text{ units}} \times X}{\cancel{150 \text{ units}}} = \frac{6 \; \cancel{\text{units}}/\text{hour} \times 150 \text{ ml}}{150 \; \cancel{\text{units}}}$$

$$X = 6 \text{ ml/hour}$$

- To administer 6 units/hour of the prescribed insulin, you need to set the infusion pump's flow rate at 6 ml/hour.

Electrolyte and nutrient infusions

- I.V. fluids can be used to deliver electrolytes and nutrients directly into the patient's bloodstream.
- Large-volume infusions with additives maintain or restore hydration or electrolyte status or supply additional electrolytes, vitamins, or other nutrients.
  - Common additives include potassium chloride, vitamins B and C, and trace elements.
  - Potassium is only added to a solution in the pharmacy; it's never added to a solution on the floor.
- Electrolytes may also be given in small-volume intermittent infusions piggybacked into existing I.V. lines.

There's nothing like a large infusion of iced tea on a warm summer's day!

- If two additives are to be added to a solution, always check the compatibility chart or consult the pharmacist to make sure that they can be safely mixed.
- If you must prepare your own additive solution, use the proportion method to calculate the amount of additive needed, and then determine the flow rate and drip rate.

> Piggybacking a small-volume electrolyte solution is really pretty easy when you know what to do.

> And a lot of fun. Hey, nice view from up here!

Calculating piggyback infusions

An I.V. piggyback is a small-volume, intermittent infusion that's connected to an existing I.V. line containing maintenance fluid.

Most piggybacks contain antibiotics or electrolytes. To calculate piggyback infusions, use proportions.

Piggyback problem

You receive an order for 500 mg of imipenem in 100 ml of normal saline solution to be infused over 1 hour. The imipenem vial contains 1,000 mg (1 g). The insert says to reconstitute the powder with 5 ml of normal saline solution. How much solution should you draw? What's the flow rate?

Calculating piggyback infusions *(continued)*

Solution solution
• Write the first ratio to describe the known solution strength (amount of drug compared to the known amount of solution):

$$1,000 \text{ mg} : 5 \text{ ml}$$

• Write the second ratio, which compares the desired dose of imipenem and the unknown amount of solution:

$$500 \text{ mg} : X$$

• Put these ratios into a proportion:

$$1,000 \text{ mg} : 5 \text{ ml} :: 500 \text{ mg} : X$$

• Multiply the extremes and the means:

$$1,000 \text{ mg} \times X = 500 \text{ mg} \times 5 \text{ ml}$$

• Solve for X by dividing each side of the equation by 1,000 mg and canceling units that appear in both the numerator and denominator:

$$\frac{\cancel{1,000 \text{ mg}} \times X}{\cancel{1,000 \text{ mg}}} = \frac{500 \cancel{\text{ mg}} \times 5 \text{ ml}}{1,000 \cancel{\text{ mg}}}$$

$$X = \frac{500 \times 5 \text{ ml}}{1,000}$$

$$X = \frac{2,500 \text{ ml}}{1,000}$$

$$X = 2.5 \text{ ml}$$

You should draw 2.5 ml of solution to get 500 mg of imipenem.

Flow rate
Recall that the flow rate is the number of milliliters of fluid to administer over 1 hour. So, in this case, the flow rate is 100 ml/hour.

Compatibility counts
After you've calculated an I.V. piggyback dose, make sure that the drugs to be infused together are compatible. The same goes for drugs mixed in the same syringe or I.V. bag. Drug compatibility charts can be time-savers—you should have one hanging in your unit's medication room. If not, use a drug handbook that includes a compatibility chart.

Learn by example

Your patient requires 1,000 ml of D_5W with 150 mg of thiamine/L over 12 hours. The thiamine is available in a prepared syringe of 100 mg/ml. How many milliliters of thiamine must be added to the solution? What's the flow rate?

- Write the first ratio to describe the known solution strength (amount of drug per 1 ml):

$$100 \text{ mg} : 1 \text{ ml}$$

- Set up the second ratio with the amount of thiamine ordered on one side and the unknown amount to be added to the solution on the other side:

$$150 \text{ mg} : X$$

- Put these ratios into a proportion:

$$100 \text{ mg} : 1 \text{ ml} :: 150 \text{ mg} : X$$

- Solve for X by multiplying the extremes and the means:

$$X \times 100 \text{ mg} = 150 \text{ mg} \times 1 \text{ ml}$$

- Divide each side of the equation by 100 mg, and cancel units that appear in both the numerator and denominator:

$$\frac{X \times \cancel{100 \text{ mg}}}{\cancel{100 \text{ mg}}} = \frac{150 \cancel{\text{mg}} \times 1 \text{ ml}}{100 \cancel{\text{mg}}}$$

$$X = \frac{150 \text{ ml}}{100}$$

$$X = 1.5 \text{ ml}$$

- You must add 1.5 ml of thiamine to the solution. If the flow rate is 1,000 ml over 12 hours, divide 1,000 by 12 to find the flow rate for 1 hour:

$$\frac{1,000 \text{ ml}}{12 \text{ hour}} = \frac{83.3 \text{ ml}}{\text{hour}}$$

- The flow rate is 83 ml/hour.

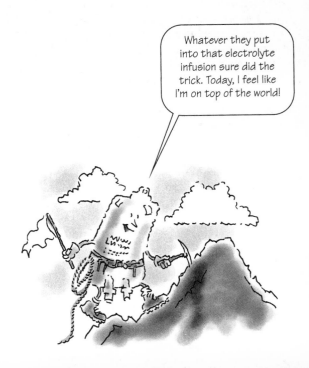

Total parenteral nutrition infusions

- Parenteral nutrition is used when nutritional needs can't be met enterally due to elevated requirements or impaired digestion or absorption in the GI tract.
  - TPN refers to any nutrient solution, including lipids, given through a central venous line.
  - Peripheral parenteral nutrition (PPN)—another form of supplemental nutrition—is administered through veins of the arms, legs, and scalp; it provides full calorie needs, but avoids the risk of a central line.
- Most facilities have a protocol regarding insertion sites and recommended solutions for TPN and PPN.
- TPN is commercially prepared or individually formulated in the pharmacy.
  - Solutions are prepared under sterile conditions to guard against patient infection.
  - Nurses rarely prepare TPN solutions on the unit.

> Sometimes, patients can't tolerate oral feedings or have impaired digestion or absorption in the GI tract. That's when they need parenteral nutrition, like TPN or PPN.

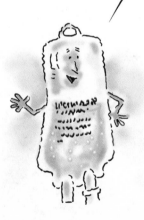

- TPN solutions contain 10% or greater dextrose concentration.
  - Amino acids are added to maintain or restore nitrogen balance.
  - Vitamins, electrolytes, and trace minerals are added to meet the patient's needs.
  - Lipids may be added, but are usually given as a separate infusion.
- TPN should be administered with an infusion pump.
- TPN is initially infused at a slow rate and then gradually increased to a maintenance dose. The rate is gradually decreased before discontinuing the TPN.
- When assessing the amount of fluid remaining in a TPN bottle, keep in mind that there may be 20 to 50 ml more than expected. (Additives increase a solution's total volume.)

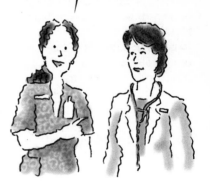

The prescriber orders the correct TPN formula based on the patient's needs.

Blood and blood product infusions

- Transfusion of blood or blood products requires the use of special equipment to prevent cell damage and maintain an adequate blood flow.
  - Blood transfusion administration sets contain a filter to remove agglutinated cells.
  - The drop factor for these sets is usually 10 to 15 gtt/ml.
- Each facility has a policy for infusing blood and blood products. Always check the policy before administering any blood or blood product.
- In general, a unit of whole blood (500 ml) or of packed red blood cells (RBCs) (250 ml) should transfuse in less than 4 hours because the blood can deteriorate and become contaminated with bacteria.

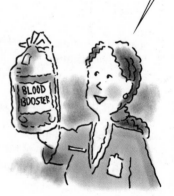

Always follow your facility's policy for transfusing blood or blood products— including using the right equipment and transfusing within the specified time.

Learn by example

Your patient is to receive 250 ml of packed RBCs over 4 hours. The drop factor of the tubing is 10 gtt/ml. What's the drip rate in drops per minute?

- First, find the flow rate in milliliters per minute:

$$\frac{250 \text{ ml of packed RBCs}}{4 \text{ hours}} = \frac{62.5 \text{ ml}}{1 \text{ hour}}$$

$$\frac{62.5 \text{ ml}}{1 \text{ hour}} \times \frac{1 \text{ hour}}{60 \text{ minutes}} = 1.04 \text{ ml/minute} = \text{flow rate}$$

- Now, multiply the flow rate by the drop factor to find the drip rate in drops per minute:

$$\frac{1.04 \text{ ml}}{1 \text{ minute}} \times \frac{10 \text{ gtt}}{1 \text{ ml}} = 10.4 \text{ gtt/minute}$$

- The drip rate is 10.4 gtt/minute, or approximately 10 gtt/minute.

Sample calculations

These problems are typical of the infusion calculations you're likely to encounter.

Calculating an erythromycin drip rate

Your patient needs 15 ml of erythromycin, which is equal to 500 mg. The infusion is to be completed in 30 minutes using a tubing set calibrated to 20 gtt/ml. What's the drip rate?

- Set up a fraction. Place the volume of the infusion in the numerator. Place the number of minutes in which the volume is to be infused in the denominator:

$$\frac{15 \text{ ml}}{30 \text{ minutes}}$$

- Multiply the fraction by the drop factor to determine the number of drops per minute to be infused (solve for X). Cancel units that appear in both the numerator and denominator:

$$X = \frac{15 \text{ ml}}{30 \text{ minutes}} \times \frac{20 \text{ gtt}}{\text{ml}}$$

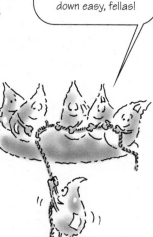

This calibration business can get a little tricky sometimes. Let him down easy, fellas!

• Solve for X by dividing the numerator by the denominator:

$$\frac{15 \times 20 \text{ gtt}}{30 \text{ minutes}}$$

$$X = \frac{300 \text{ gtt}}{30 \text{ minutes}}$$

$$X = 10 \text{ gtt/minute}$$

• The drip rate is 10 gtt/minute.

Calculating a lactated Ringer's infusion time

If you infuse 1,050 ml of lactated Ringer's solution at 25 gtt/minute using a set calibration of 10 gtt/ml, what's the infusion time?

• Use the information you know to set up the formula:

$$X = \frac{1,050 \text{ ml}}{(25 \text{ gtt/minute} \div 10 \text{ gtt/ml}) \times 60 \text{ minutes}}$$

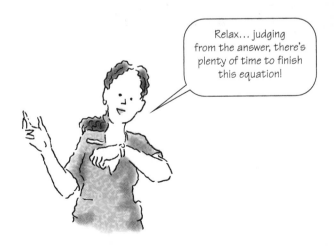

Relax... judging from the answer, there's plenty of time to finish this equation!

- Divide the drip rate by the drop factor. (Remember to multiply the dividend by the reciprocal of the divisor). Cancel units that appear in both the numerator and denominator:

$$\frac{25 \text{ gtt}}{1 \text{ min}} \times \frac{1 \text{ ml}}{10 \text{ gtt}} = 2.5 \text{ ml/minute}$$

- Rewrite the equation (solving for X) using the result (2.5 ml/minute) in the denominator. Cancel units that appear in both the numerator and denominator:

$$X = \frac{1,050 \text{ ml}}{\dfrac{2.5 \text{ ml}}{1 \text{ min}} \times \dfrac{60 \text{ min}}{1 \text{ hour}}}$$

- To find the infusion time, solve for X:

$$X = \frac{1,050}{2.5 \times 60 \text{ hours}}$$

$$X = \frac{1,050}{150 \text{ hours}}$$

- Divide the numerator by the denominator:

$$X = 7 \text{ hours}$$

- The infusion time is 7 hours.

Special calculations

7

Sometimes, you need different calculations when working in specialty departments. This chapter covers the calculations you'll use in pediatric, obstetric, and critical care areas.

Pediatric drugs

- Because of their size, metabolism, and other factors, children have different medication needs than adults.
  - A child's immature body systems may be unable to handle certain drugs.
  - A child has a greater proportion of water, which alters drug distribution.
- Calculating pediatric dosages requires special care.

> Let's face it... I'm small, but I have enormous needs. When you're giving medications, please remember to treat me with kid gloves!

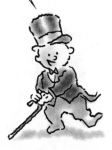

Help desk

A trio of time-saving tips

When calculating safe pediatric dosages, save time and stop errors by following these suggestions:
- Carry a calculator for use when solving equations.
- Consult a formulary or drug handbook to verify a drug dose. When in doubt, call the pharmacist.
- Keep your patient's weight in kilograms at his bedside so you don't have to estimate it or weigh him in a rush.

- To verify the safety of a pediatric drug dosage, use the dosage-per-kilogram-of-body weight method or the body surface area (BSA) method; other methods are less accurate for children.

Administering drugs to pediatric patients

- Although children receive drugs by the same routes as adults, they require different methods of administration.
- Each route has specific administration guidelines and precautions.

Help desk

Giving medications to children

When giving oral and parenteral medications to children, safety is essential. Keep these points in mind:
- Check the child's mouth to make sure that he has swallowed the oral drug.
- Carefully mix oral drugs that come in suspension form.
- Give I.M. injections in the vastus lateralis muscle of infants who haven't started walking.
- Don't inject more than 1 ml into I.M. or subcutaneous sites.
- Rotate injection sites.

Oral route

- Infants and young children who can't swallow tablets are given oral drugs in liquid form.
  - If a liquid form isn't available, most tablets can be crushed and mixed in a liquid.
  - Don't try to administer medications in essential fluids, such as breast milk or formula, because this may lead to feeding refusal.
  - Only mix in a small amount of liquid so the child is more likely to finish it.

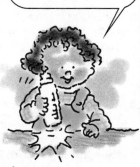

I'm onto that old sneak-the-medicine-into-the-baby bottle trick... so don't even think about it!

- If a child can drink from a cup, measure and give liquid medications in a cup that's calibrated in metric and household units. If he can't drink from a cup, use a medication dropper, syringe, or hollow-handle spoon.
- Mix all liquid suspensions thoroughly before measuring and administering them.
- After giving an oral drug, check the child's mouth to make sure that the entire drug was swallowed.

Subcutaneous route

- Some medications, such as certain immunizations and insulin, may be given subcutaneously (subQ).
- A subQ injection should contain no more than 1 ml of solution.
- Any area with sufficient subcutaneous tissue may be used—the upper arm, abdomen, and thigh are the most common.

I.M. route

- Many vaccines are commonly administered intramuscularly.
- Each injection should contain no more than 1 ml of solution.

I.M. injections for infants

When giving I.M. injections to infants, use the vastus lateralis muscle. Don't inject into the gluteus muscle until it's fully developed, which occurs when the child learns to walk. Use a 23G to 25G needle that's $5/8''$ to $1''$ in length. These illustrations show how to give an I.M. injection using one- and two-person methods.

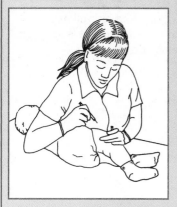 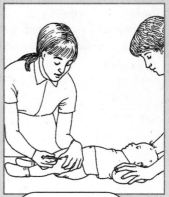

- Infants should receive I.M. injections in their thighs and not their gluteal muscles.

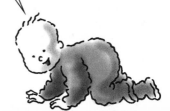

Which muscle you use for an injection will depend on whether I can walk. As you can see, my gluteus maximus still has a way to go.

I.V. route

- Fluids and various drugs may be administered I.V.—through either a peripheral or central vein.
- Because children can tolerate only a limited amount of fluid, be sure to dilute I.V. drugs and administer I.V. fluids cautiously.
- Always use an infusion pump with infants and small children.
- Check the I.V. site before giving the fluid as well as during and after administration; children's blood vessels are immature and can be easily damaged by drugs.

Topical route

- Children absorb topical medications at a higher rate than adults due to their:
  – thinner stratum corneum
  – increased skin hydration
  – greater ratio of total BSA to weight.
- Be aware that the plastic lining of a disposable diaper acts like an occlusive dressing and can increase the absorption rate of drugs applied to the diaper area.

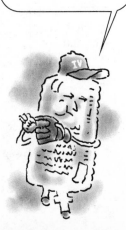

Don't take chances with your future all-star's pitching arm! Always check the I.V. site for signs of inflammation or infiltration before, during, and after drug administration.

Calculating dosages
(based on kilograms of body weight)

- The most accurate and common way to calculate pediatric doses is to use the dosage-per-kilogram-of-body weight method.
- Most drug companies provide information about safe doses for pediatric patients in milligrams per kilogram of body weight—usually expressed as mg/kg/day or mg/kg/dose.
- You can determine the pediatric dose by multiplying the child's weight in kilograms by the required number of milligrams of drug per kilogram.

For this calculation method, you need to have an accurate measure of the child's weight. Be sure to use a scale that's appropriate for the patient's size, and check that it's properly calibrated.

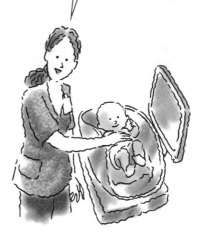

Learn by example

The prescriber orders a single dose of 20 mg/kg/dose of amoxicillin oral suspension for a toddler who weighs 20 lb (9.1 kg). What's the dose in milligrams?

- Set up the proportion with the ordered dosage in one fraction and the unknown dosage and the patient's weight in the other fraction:

$$\frac{20 \text{ mg}}{1 \text{ kg/dose}} = \frac{X}{9 \text{ kg/dose}}$$

- Cross-multiply the fractions:

$$X \times 1 \text{ kg/dose} = 20 \text{ mg} \times 9 \text{ kg/dose}$$

- Solve for X by dividing each side of the equation by 1 kg/dose and canceling units that appear in both the numerator and denominator:

$$\frac{X \times 1 \ \cancel{\text{kg/dose}}}{1 \ \cancel{\text{kg/dose}}} = \frac{20 \text{ mg} \times 9 \ \cancel{\text{kg/dose}}}{1 \ \cancel{\text{kg/dose}}}$$

$$X = 180 \text{ mg}$$

- The patient needs 180 mg of amoxicillin.

> Check your math carefully... an error can have weighty consequences for your pediatric patient.

Learn by example

The prescriber orders penicillin V potassium oral suspension 56 mg/kg/day in four divided doses for a patient who weighs 55 lb. The suspension that's available is penicillin V potassium 125 mg/5 ml. What volume should you administer for each dose?

- First, convert the child's weight from pounds to kilograms by setting up a proportion:

$$X : 55 \text{ lb} :: 1 \text{ kg} : 2.2 \text{ lb}$$

- Multiply the means and the extremes:

$$X \times 2.2 \text{ lb} = 1 \text{ kg} \times 55 \text{ lb}$$

- Solve for X by dividing each side of the equation by 2.2 lb and canceling units that appear in both the numerator and denominator:

$$\frac{X \times \cancel{2.2 \text{ lb}}}{\cancel{2.2 \text{ lb}}} = \frac{1 \text{ kg} \times 55 \cancel{\text{ lb}}}{2.2 \cancel{\text{ lb}}}$$

$$X = \frac{55 \text{ kg}}{2.2}$$

$$X = 25 \text{ kg}$$

> Did I hear you right... **four** whole doses of that yicky, icky stuff?

> OK, now Simon says 'Raise your extremes...'

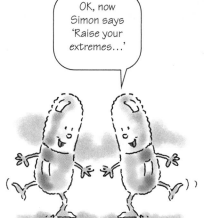

- The child weighs 25 kg. Next, determine the total daily dosage by setting up a proportion with the patient's weight and the unknown dosage on one side and the ordered dosage on the other side:

$$\frac{25 \text{ kg}}{X} = \frac{1 \text{ kg}}{56 \text{ mg}}$$

- Cross-multiply the fractions:

$$X \times 1 \text{ kg} = 56 \text{ mg} \times 25 \text{ kg}$$

- Solve for X by dividing each side of the equation by 1 kg and canceling units that appear in both the numerator and denominator:

$$\frac{X \times \cancel{1 \text{ kg}}}{1 \text{ kg}} = \frac{56 \text{ mg} \times 25 \cancel{\text{ kg}}}{1 \text{ kg}}$$

$$X = \frac{56 \text{ mg} \times 25}{1}$$

$$X = 1{,}400 \text{ mg}$$

- The child's daily dosage is 1,400 mg. Now, divide the daily dosage by 4 doses to determine the dose to administer every 6 hours:

$$X = \frac{1{,}400 \text{ mg}}{4 \text{ doses}}$$

$$X = 350 \text{ mg/dose}$$

- The child should receive 350 mg every 6 hours.
- Lastly, calculate the volume to give for each dose by set-

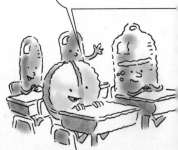

I actually like math... it's these multipart problems that always trip me up.

ting up a proportion with the unknown volume and the amount in one dose on one side and the available dose on the other side:

$$\frac{X}{350 \text{ mg}} = \frac{5 \text{ ml}}{125 \text{ mg}}$$

- Cross-multiply the fractions:

$$X \times 125 \text{ mg} = 5 \text{ ml} \times 350 \text{ mg}$$

- Solve for X by dividing each side of the equation by 125 mg and canceling units that appear in both the numerator and denominator:

$$\frac{X \times \cancel{125 \text{ mg}}}{\cancel{125 \text{ mg}}} = \frac{5 \text{ ml} \times 350 \cancel{\text{ mg}}}{125 \cancel{\text{ mg}}}$$

$$X = \frac{5 \text{ ml} \times 350}{125}$$

$$X = \frac{1,750 \text{ mg}}{125}$$

$$X = 14 \text{ ml}$$

- You should administer 14 ml of the drug at each dose.

Calculating dosages (based on BSA)

- A child's BSA may be used to calculate safe pediatric dosages for a limited number of drugs, such as antineoplastic or chemotherapeutic agents.

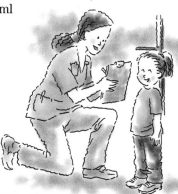

Step 1 involves measuring and plotting the patient's height and weight on a nomogram... step 2, making the necessary calculation.

- Calculating a dosage based on the BSA is done in two steps:

  ☝ Plot the patient's height and weight on a chart called a *nomogram* to determine the BSA in square meters (m^2).

  ✌ Multiply the BSA by the prescribed pediatric dose in $mg/m^2/day$ using this formula:

$$\text{child's dose in mg} = \text{child's BSA in } m^2 \times \frac{\text{pediatric dose in mg}}{m^2/\text{day}}$$

- The BSA method can also be used to calculate a child's dose based on the average adult BSA—$1.73\ m^2$—and an average adult dose of the given drug using this formula:

$$\frac{\text{child's dose}}{\text{in mg}} = \frac{\text{child's BSA in } m^2}{\text{average adult BSA } (1.73\ m^2)} \times \frac{\text{average}}{\text{adult dose}}$$

Learn by example

The prescriber orders ephedrine 100 $mg/m^2/day$ for a child who's 40″ tall and weighs 64 lb. How much ephedrine should the child receive daily?

- Use the nomogram to determine the child's BSA—in this case, $0.96\ m^2$.
- Using the appropriate formula, determine the daily dosage:

$$X = 0.96\ m^2 \times \frac{100\ \text{mg}}{1\ m^2/\text{day}}$$

- Solve for X:

$$X = 0.96\ \cancel{m^2} \times \frac{100\ \text{mg}}{1\ \cancel{m^2}/\text{day}}$$

$$X = 96\ \text{mg/day}$$

- The child needs 96 mg of ephedrine per day.

What's in a nomogram?

Body surface area (BSA) is critical when calculating dosages for pediatric patients or for drugs that are extremely potent and need to be given in precise amounts. The nomogram shown here lets you plot the patient's height and weight to determine the BSA. Here's how it works:
• Locate the patient's height in the left column of the nomogram and his weight in the right column.
• Use a ruler to draw a straight line connecting the two points. The point where the line intersects the surface area column indicates the patient's BSA in square meters.
• For an average-size child, use the simplified nomogram in the box. Just find the child's weight in pounds on the left side of the scale, and then read the corresponding BSA on the right side.

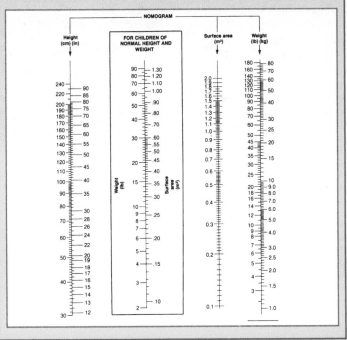

Learn by example

A child who needs chemotherapy is 36″ tall and weighs 40 lb. What's the safe drug dose if the average adult dose is 1,000 mg?

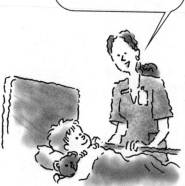

> Remember, you can calculate a pediatric dose by dividing the child's BSA by the average adult BSA and multiplying that number by the average adult dose of the drug.

• Use the nomogram to determine the child's BSA—in this case, 0.72 m².

• Then set up an equation using the appropriate formula. Divide the child's BSA by 1.73 m² (the average adult BSA), and multiply by the average adult dose, which is 1,000 mg:

$$X = \frac{0.72 \text{ m}^2}{1.73 \text{ m}^2} \times 1,000 \text{ mg}$$

• Now, solve for X by canceling units that appear in both the numerator and denominator, multiplying the child's BSA by the average adult dose, and dividing the result by the average adult BSA:

$$X = \frac{0.72 \cancel{\text{m}^2} \times 1,000 \text{ mg}}{1.73 \cancel{\text{m}^2}}$$

$$X = 416 \text{ mg}$$

• The safe dose for this child is 416 mg.

Verifying calculations

- The nurse is the "last line of defense" in verifying that the ordered dosage is safe.
- There are several ways to verify that your calculation is correct, including:
  - consulting a nursing drug handbook, which typically contains the recommended pediatric dosages for commonly prescribed drugs
  - asking the pharmacist to verify that the dosage is correct
  - asking another nurse to double-check your math (always do this for complex calculations).

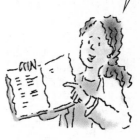

One easy way to verify your calculation is to look up the dosage in a reliable nursing drug handbook.

Administering I.V. fluids

- I.V. drugs and fluids can be given by either continuous or intermittent infusion to pediatric patients.
- Follow all written guidelines and protocols for dosages, fluid volumes for dilution, and administration rates.
- Children's fluid needs are proportionally greater than adults.
  - Extracellular fluid has a higher percentage of water, so fluid exchange rates are two to three times higher for children than adults, making them more susceptible to dehydration.
  - You can calculate the number of milliliters of fluid a child needs based on weight in kilograms, metabolism (calories required), and BSA in square meters.

Continuous infusions

- These infusions are used when a patient requires around-the-clock fluids or drug therapy or both.
- Fluids may be used to maintain volume or to correct an existing fluid or electrolyte imbalance.
- To prepare the infusion, add the drug to a small-volume bag of I.V. fluid or a volume-control device.
  - Always follow the manufacturer's guidelines for mixing the solutions carefully.
  - Remember that pediatric patients can only tolerate small amounts of fluid.
- There are five steps to starting a continuous infusion:

  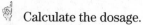 Calculate the dosage.

  Draw up the drug in a syringe, and then add the drug to the I.V. bag or fluid chamber through the drug-additive port using aseptic technique.

  Mix the drug thoroughly.

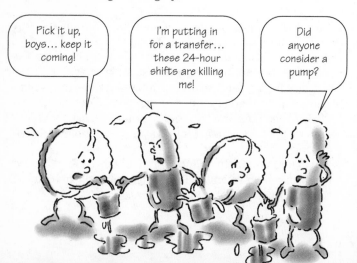

Label the I.V. bag or fluid chamber with the drug's name, dosage, time and date it was mixed, and your initials.

Hang the solution and administer the drug by infusion pump at the prescribed flow rate.

Intermittent infusions
- These infusions are used when drugs or fluids need to be administered periodically.
  - A vascular access device is kept in place, eliminating the need for continuous fluid infusion.
  - The child can remain mobile, minimizing the potential for volume overload.
- Volume-control devices have 100- to 150-ml fluid chambers calibrated in 1-ml increments; medication-filled syringes with microtubing can also be used to infuse small volumes via syringe pumps.

I.V. infusion control

Accurate fluid administration is extremely important for pediatric patients. So, syringes, infusion pumps, and other volume-control devices are used extensively to regulate continuous and intermittent I.V. infusions. One typical device, the Buretrol set, is shown here.

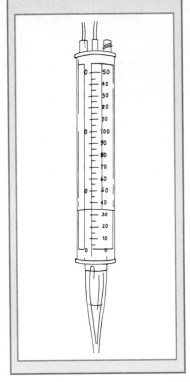

- The I.V. infusion rate must be carefully controlled to ensure proper absorption and to prevent or minimize toxicity associated with rapid infusion.

It's nice to have a little time off now and then!

- There are 10 steps to starting an intermittent infusion with a volume-control device:

👆 Carefully calculate the prescribed volume of the drug. (Be aware that some facilities consider the drug volume as part of the diluent volume.)

✌️ Draw up the prescribed volume of the drug into the syringe.

👌 Add the drug to the fluid chamber through the drug-additive port, using aseptic technique.

🖐️ Mix the drug thoroughly.

🖐️ Attach the volume-control device to an electronic infusion pump to control the infusion rate. If you're using a small-volume I.V. bag instead of a volume-control device and pump, use microdrip tubing, which has a drop factor of 60 gtt/ml.

🖐️🖐️ Calculate the appropriate flow rate, and infuse the drug.

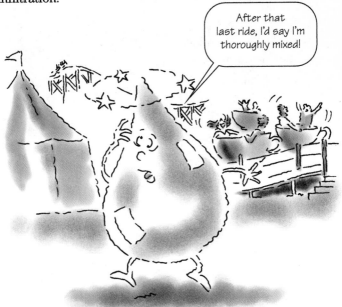 Label the volume-control device with the name of the drug.

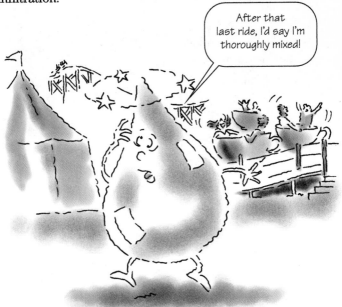 When the infusion is complete, flush the line to clear the tubing. Administer the flush at the same rate as the drug, and label the volume-control device to indicate that the flush is infusing.

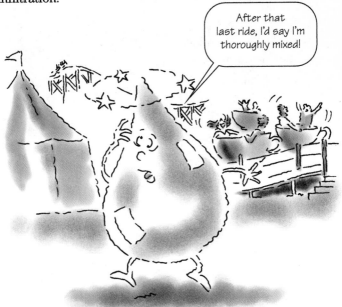 With an intermittent infusion, disconnect the device when the flush is complete.

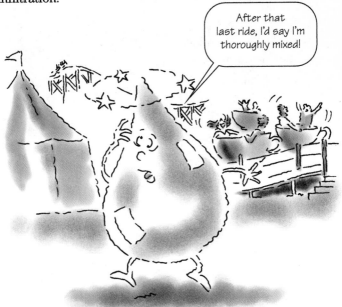 During the infusion, check the I.V. site frequently for infiltration.

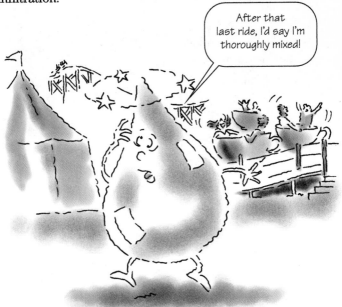

Calculating fluid needs (based on weight)

- Three different formulas can be used to calculate fluid needs, depending on the child's weight.

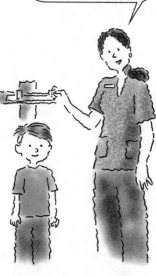

Make sure that you have an accurate weight before using this calculation method.

- A child weighing less than 10 kg requires 100 ml of fluid per kilogram of body weight.
  - Convert the child's weight from pounds to kilograms, and then multiply by 100 ml/kg/day.
  - Use this formula:

Weight in kg × 100 ml/kg/day = Fluid needs in ml/day

- A child weighing 10 to 20 kg needs 1,000 ml of fluid per day for the first 10 kg plus 50 ml for every kilogram over 10.
  - Convert the weight from pounds to kilograms.
  - Subtract 10 kg from the child's total weight, and then multiply the result by 50 mg/kg/day.
  - Here's the formula:

(total kg − 10 kg) × 50 ml/kg/day = additional fluid needed in ml/day

  - Add the additional daily fluid to the 1,000 ml/day required for the first 10 kg for the child's daily fluid requirement:

1,000 ml/day + Additional fluid needed = Fluid needs in ml/day

- A child weighing more than 20 kg requires 1,500 ml of fluid for the first 20 kg plus 20 ml for each additional kilogram.

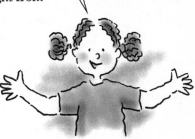

Don't forget to convert from pounds to kilograms. It makes a big difference!

  - Convert the child's weight from pounds to kilograms.
  - Subtract 20 kg from the child's total weight, and then multiply the result by 20 ml/kg to find the child's additional fluid needs.
  - Use this formula:

$$(\text{total kg} - 20 \text{ kg}) \times 20 \text{ ml/kg/day} = \text{additional fluid needed in ml/day}$$

  - Because the child needs 1,500 ml of fluid per day for the first 20 kg, add the additional fluid needed to 1,500 ml. The total is the child's daily fluid requirement:

$$1{,}500 \text{ ml/day} + \text{Additional fluid needed} = \text{Fluid needs in ml/day}$$

Learn by example

How much fluid should you give a 44-lb patient over 24 hours to meet his maintenance needs?

- First, convert 44 lb to kilograms by setting up a proportion with fractions:

$$\frac{44 \text{ lb}}{X} = \frac{2.2 \text{ lb}}{1 \text{ kg}}$$

- Cross-multiply the fractions, and then solve for X by dividing both sides of the equation by 2.2 lb and canceling units that appear in both the numerator and denominator:

$$X \times 2.2 \text{ lb} = 44 \text{ lb} \times 1 \text{ kg}$$

$$\frac{X \times \cancel{2.2 \text{ lb}}}{\cancel{2.2 \text{ lb}}} = \frac{44 \cancel{\text{ lb}} \times 1 \text{ kg}}{2.2 \cancel{\text{ lb}}}$$

$$X = \frac{44 \text{ kg}}{2.2}$$

$$X = 20 \text{ kg}$$

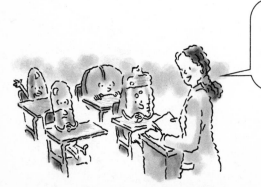

Would anyone like to try solving this problem on the blackboard for the whole class?

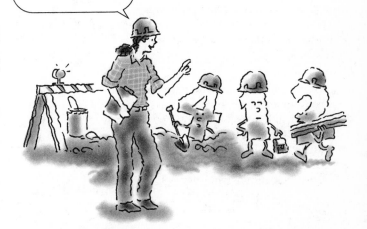

- The child weighs 20 kg. Now, subtract 10 kg from the child's weight and multiply the result by 50 ml/kg/day to find the child's additional fluid needs:

$$X = (20 \text{ kg} - 10 \text{ kg}) \times 50 \text{ ml/kg/day}$$

$$X = 10 \cancel{\text{ kg}} \times 50 \text{ ml/}\cancel{\text{kg}}\text{/day}$$

$$X = 500 \text{ ml/day additional fluid needed}$$

- Next, add the additional fluid needed to the 1,000 ml/day required for the first 10 kg:

$$X = 1,000 \text{ ml/day} + 500 \text{ ml/day}$$

$$X = 1,500 \text{ ml/day}$$

- The child should receive 1,500 ml of fluid in 24 hours to meet his fluid maintenance needs.

Calculating fluid needs (based on calories)

- Fluid needs can be based on calories because water is needed for metabolism.
- A child should receive 120 ml of fluid for every 100 kilocalories (kcal) of metabolism.
- Follow these steps to calculate fluid requirements based on calorie requirements:
  - Find the child's calorie requirement. Use a table of recommended dietary allowances, or ask a dietitian to calculate it.
  - Divide the calorie requirements by 100 kcal, because fluid requirements are determined for every 100 calories.
  - Multiply the results by 120 ml, the amount of fluid required for every 100 kcal.
  - Here's the formula:

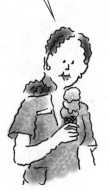

What? It meets my daily-recommended dietary needs. Besides, it isn't even real ice cream... it's one of those fat-free varieties. Hardly any calories at all!

$$\text{fluid requirement in ml/day} = \frac{\text{calorie requirements}}{100 \text{ kcal}} \times 120 \text{ ml}$$

Learn by example

Your pediatric patient uses 900 calories/day. What are her daily fluid requirements?

- Set up the formula, inserting the appropriate numbers and substituting X for the unknown amount of fluid.

$$X = \frac{900 \text{ kcal}}{100 \text{ kcal}} \times 120 \text{ ml}$$

$$X = 9 \times 120 \text{ ml}$$

$$X = 1{,}080 \text{ ml}$$

- The patient needs 1,080 ml of fluid per day.

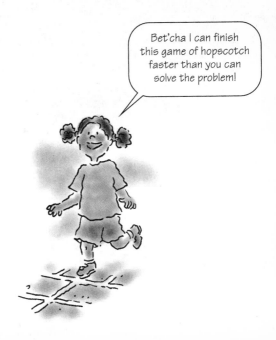

Bet'cha I can finish this game of hopscotch faster than you can solve the problem!

Calculating fluid needs (based on BSA)

- This calculation method may be used for children who aren't dehydrated.
- Simply multiply the BSA by 1,500 using this formula:

$$\text{Fluid maintenance needed in ml/day} = \text{BSA in m}^2 \times 1{,}500 \text{ ml/day/m}^2$$

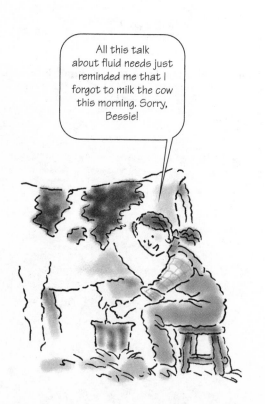

Learn by example

Your patient is 36″ tall and weighs 40 lb (18.1 kg). If his BSA is 0.72 m², how much fluid does he need each day?

- Set up the equation, inserting the appropriate numbers and substituting X for the unknown amount of fluid. Then solve for X.

$$X = 0.72 \; \cancel{m^2} \times 1{,}500 \; ml/day/\cancel{m^2}$$

$$X = 1{,}080 \; ml/day$$

- The child needs 1,080 ml of fluid per day.

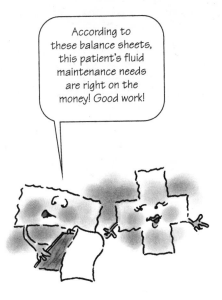

According to these balance sheets, this patient's fluid maintenance needs are right on the money! Good work!

Obstetric drugs

- During pregnancy, labor and delivery, and the postpartum period, drugs are commonly given for four reasons:

   to control gestational hypertension

   to inhibit preterm labor

   to induce labor

   to prevent postpartum hemorrhage.

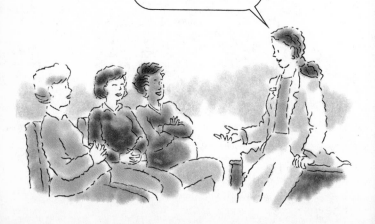

I know you're all anticipating a natural childbirth experience, but you need to know about the medications that are commonly given for special situations.

- When administering medication, you need to frequently check the mother's vital signs, urine output, uterine contractions, and deep tendon reflexes.
- It's also important to carefully assess intake and output and breath sounds to reduce the risk of fluid overload.

Assessing the mother's body systems

Assessment is a critical part of obstetric nursing. Here's what to assess in each of the mother's body systems.

Neurologic system
- Deep tendon reflexes when magnesium sulfate is infusing
- Pain
- Orientation (because disorientation can indicate hypoxemia or water intoxication)

Cardiovascular system
- Vital signs
- Extremities for peripheral edema with large-volume infusions
- Pulses and skin temperature in the lower extremities for evidence of deep vein thrombosis; also for Homans' sign by dorsiflexing the foot while supporting the leg (deep calf pain may indicate thrombophlebitis)
- I.V. site to prevent infiltration

Respiratory system
- Breath sounds
- Need for oxygen
- Lungs for pulmonary edema with large-volume infusions

GI system
- Abdomen for contractions when oxytocin is infusing
- Abdomen for bowel sounds after delivery
- Ability to pass flatus or move bowels before discharge

Genitourinary system
- Urine output
- Fluid balance to check for decreased renal function

- It's equally important to evaluate the fetus's response to drug therapy.
  - Assess fetal heart tone and heart rate.
  - Stay alert for a sudden increase or decrease in fetal heart rate.

It's got a good beat: Contractions and fetal heart rate

Electronic fetal monitoring allows you to assess the mother's contractions as well as the fetal heart rate (FHR). Follow these steps.

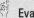 Evaluate the mother's contraction pattern.

 Note the characteristics of the contractions.
- What's the frequency?
- What's the duration?
- What's the intensity?

 Evaluate the FHR after establishing a baseline.
- Is the rate within normal range?
- Is tachycardia present?
- Is bradycardia present?

 Determine the FHR variability.
- What's the short-term variability (only with internal fetal monitoring)?
- What's the long-term variability?

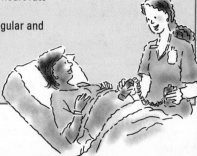 Assess for changes in FHR characteristics.
- Is acceleration or increased heart rate present with contractions?
- Is deceleration or decreased heart rate present with contractions?
- Is the heart rate waveform regular and uniform in shape?
- Is the heart rate waveform irregular in shape?

Just checking the baby's heart rate... everything seems to be whooshing along fine!

Commonly administered drugs

Four drugs are commonly used during pregnancy, labor and delivery, and the postpartum period:

- terbutaline
- magnesium sulfate
- dinoprostone
- oxytocin.

Terbutaline

- This drug inhibits preterm labor by stimulating beta$_2$-adrenergic receptors in the uterine smooth muscle, thereby inhibiting contractility.
- To administer, mix in a compatible I.V. solution by infusion pump.
- Titrate the dose every 10 minutes until the contractions subside, the maximum dose is reached, or the patient can't tolerate the adverse effects.

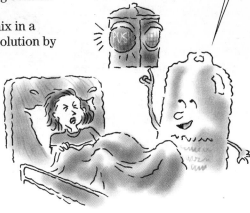

Depending on the circumstances, some obstetric drugs will tell the body when to stop contractions... others when to start. Looks like we're a "go"!

Magnesium sulfate

- This drug prevents or controls seizures that may be caused by gestational hypertension.
- To administer, first give a loading dose and then follow with an infusion at a lower dose, as prescribed.
- During the infusion, closely assess knee jerk and patellar reflexes. Loss of these reflexes signal drug toxicity.
- If toxicity is suspected, immediately stop the infusion and notify the practitioner.

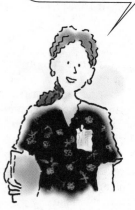

If magnesium sulfate is ordered, monitor your patient's reflexes closely for signs of toxicity.

Dinoprostone

- This drug is used to induce labor by opening the cervix in pregnant patients who are at or near term.
- It's available as an endocervical gel, vaginal insert, or vaginal suppository.
- Be aware that administration of this drug doesn't fall within the scope of practice for nurses in all states.
- To administer, have the patient lie on her back. Using aseptic technique, the practitioner will insert the gel into the cervical canal.

Oxytocin

- This drug is most commonly used to induce labor.
- Mix with a compatible I.V. solution and administer via piggyback with an infusion pump, titrating until a normal contraction pattern occurs.
- The dose may be decreased when labor is firmly established.
- Carefully monitor the strength of contractions. Severe contractions that can lead to uterine rupture may occur.

Dosage calculations

- Administering accurate dosages to the mother helps avoid fetal complications.
- Examine all drug labels closely.

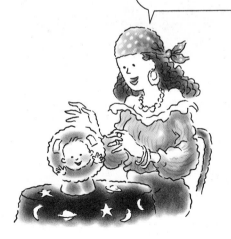

Yes, I see a baby in your immediate future... sometime within the next few hours, if I'm not mistaken!

(Text continues on page 244.)

Dodging drug dangers

The lowdown on four obstetric drugs

This table lists some common drugs used in the obstetric setting along with their actions, adverse reactions, and nursing considerations.

Drug	Action	Adverse reactions
terbutaline	Relaxes uterine muscle by acting on beta$_2$-adrenergic receptors; inhibits uterine contractions	**Maternal** • *Blood:* increased liver enzymes • *Central nervous system (CNS):* seizures, nervousness, tremor, headache, drowsiness, flushing, sweating • *Cardiovascular:* increased heart rate, changes in blood pressure, palpitations, chest discomfort • *Eye, ear, nose, and throat (EENT):* tinnitus • *GI:* nausea, vomiting, altered taste • *Respiratory:* dyspnea, wheezing
magnesium sulfate	May decrease acetylcholine released by nerve impulse, but anti-convulsant mechanisms unknown	**Maternal** • *CNS:* sweating, drowsiness, depressed reflexes, flaccid paralysis, hypothermia, flushing, blurred vision • *Cardiovascular:* hypotension, circulatory collapse, depressed cardiac function, heart block • *Other:* fatal respiratory paralysis, hypocalcemia with tetany

Nursing considerations

• Use cautiously in the patient with diabetes, hypertension, hyperthyroidism, severe cardiac disease, and arrhythmias.
• Protect the drug from light. Don't use if it's discolored.
• Explain the need for the drug to the patient and her family.
• Give subcutaneous injection in lateral deltoid area.
• Warn the patient about the possibility of paradoxical bronchospasm.
• Tell the patient she may use tablets and aerosol concomitantly.
• Tell the patient how to administer a metered dose.
• Although not approved by the Food and Drug Administration for treatment of preterm labor, this drug is considered very effective and is used in many hospitals.
• Monitor the neonate for hypoglycemia.
• Monitor the patient's blood glucose level with long-term use.

• Use cautiously in labor and in those with impaired renal function, myocardial damage, or heart block.
• This drug may be used as a tocolytic agent to inhibit premature labor; it can decrease the frequency and force of uterine contractions.
• Keep calcium gluconate available to reverse magnesium sulfate intoxication.
• Use cautiously in the patient undergoing digitalization because arrhythmias may occur.
• Watch for respiratory depression.
• Monitor intake and output.

(continued)

The lowdown on four obstetric drugs *(continued)*

Drug	Action	Adverse reactions
magnesium sulfate *(continued)*		
dinoprostone	Produces strong, prompt contractions of uterine smooth muscle; facilitates cervical dilation by directly softening the cervix	**Maternal** • *CNS:* fever, headache, dizziness, anxiety, paresthesia, weakness, syncope • *Cardiovascular:* chest pain, arrhythmias • *EENT:* blurred vision, eye pain • *GI:* nausea, vomiting, diarrhea • *Genitourinary:* vaginal pain, vaginitis, endometritis **Fetal** • *CNS:* hypotonia, hyperstimulation • *Respiratory:* respiratory depression • *Cardiovascular:* bradycardia • *Other:* intrauterine fetal sepsis
oxytocin	Causes potent and selective stimulation of uterine and mammary gland smooth muscle	**Maternal** • *Blood:* afibrinogenemia (may be from postpartum bleeding) • *CNS:* subarachnoid hemorrhage resulting from hypertension; seizures or coma resulting from water intoxication

Nursing considerations

- Monitor deep tendon reflexes.
- Maximum infusion is 150 mg/minute.
- Signs of hypermagnesemia begin to appear at blood levels of 4 mEq/L.
- This drug should be stopped at least 2 hours before delivery to avoid fetal respiratory depression.
- Monitor the neonate for magnesium sulfate toxicity.

- Use only with the patient in or near a delivery suite. Critical care facilities should be available.
- After administration of the gel form of the drug, the patient should remain supine for 10 minutes.
- Have the patient remain supine for 2 hours after insertion of the vaginal insert form of the drug.
- Remove the vaginal insert with the onset of active labor or 12 hours after insertion.
- Monitor the fetus accordingly.
- If hyperstimulation of the uterus occurs, gently flush the vagina with sterile saline solution.
- Treat dinoprostone-induced fever (usually self-limiting and transient) with water sponging and increased fluid intake, not with aspirin.

- Oxytocin is contraindicated in cephalopelvic disproportion; where delivery requires conversion, as in transverse lie; in fetal distress; when delivery isn't imminent; and in other obstetric emergencies.
- Administer by piggyback infusion so the drug can be discontinued without interrupting the I.V. line. Don't give by I.V. bolus injection.
- Don't infuse in more than one site.

(continued)

The lowdown on four obstetric drugs *(continued)*

Drug	Action	Adverse reactions
oxytocin *(continued)*		• *Cardiovascular:* hypotension, increased heart rate, systemic venous return, increased cardiac output, arrhythmias • *Other:* hypersensitivity, tetanic uterine contractions, abruptio placentae, impaired uterine blood flow, increased uterine motility, uterine rupture ***Fetal*** • *Blood:* hyperbilirubinemia, hypercapnia • *Cardiovascular:* bradycardia, tachycardia, premature ventricular contractions, variable deceleration of heart rate • *Respiratory:* hypoxia, asphyxia, death • *CNS:* brain damage, seizures • *EENT:* retinal hemorrhage • *GI:* hepatic necrosis

Nursing considerations

• Monitor and record uterine contractions, heart rate, blood pressure, intrauterine pressure, fetal heart rate, and character of blood loss every 15 minutes.
• Have magnesium sulfate (20% solution) available for relaxation of myometrium.
• Monitor fluid intake and output. Antidiuretic effect may lead to fluid overload, seizures, and coma.

Looks like I'll be doing a little labor myself... piggybacking a solution to hurry the birthing process along.

Learn by example

Your patient is 10 days overdue, so the prescriber orders oxytocin to stimulate labor. The order reads *1 ml (10 units) oxytocin in 1 L (1,000 ml) NSS; infuse via pump at 2 milliunits/minute for 20 minutes and then increase flow rate to 3 milliunits/minute.* What's the solution's concentration? What's the flow rate needed to deliver 2 milliunits/minute for 20 minutes? What's the flow rate needed to deliver 3 milliunits/minute thereafter?

- Determine the concentration of the solution by setting up a proportion with the ordered concentration in one fraction and the unknown concentration in the other fraction:

$$\frac{10 \text{ units}}{1,000 \text{ ml}} = \frac{X}{1 \text{ ml}}$$

- Cross-multiply the fractions:

$$X \times 1,000 \text{ ml} = 10 \text{ units} \times 1 \text{ ml}$$

- Solve for X by dividing both sides of the equation by 1,000 ml and canceling units that appear in both the numerator and denominator:

$$\frac{X \times \cancel{1,000 \text{ ml}}}{\cancel{1,000 \text{ ml}}} = \frac{10 \text{ units} \times 1 \cancel{\text{ml}}}{1,000 \cancel{\text{ml}}}$$

$$X = \frac{10 \text{ units}}{1,000}$$

$$X = 0.01 \text{ unit}$$

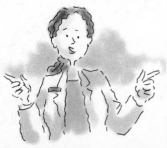

Don't forget to divide both sides of the equation by 1,000 ml and cancel like units.

- The amount 0.01 unit can be written in milliunits: 1 milliunit is 1/1,000 of a unit; 1,000 milliunits is 1 unit. Therefore, 0.01 unit times 1,000 equals 10 milliunits. So the concentration is 10 milliunits/ml.

- Next, determine the flow rate. If the prescribed dosage of oxytocin is 2 milliunits/minute for 20 minutes, the patient receives a total of 40 milliunits. To calculate the rate needed to provide that dose, set up a proportion with the known concentration in one fraction and the total oxytocin dose and unknown flow rate in the other:

$$\frac{10 \text{ milliunits}}{1 \text{ ml}} = \frac{40 \text{ milliunits}}{X}$$

- Cross-multiply the fractions:

$$X \times 10 \text{ milliunits} = 1 \text{ ml} \times 40 \text{ milliunits}$$

- Solve for X by dividing both sides of the equation by 10 milliunits and canceling units that appear in both the numerator and denominator:

$$\frac{X \times \cancel{10 \text{ milliunits}}}{\cancel{10 \text{ milliunits}}} = \frac{1 \text{ ml} \times 40 \cancel{\text{ milliunits}}}{10 \cancel{\text{ milliunits}}}$$

$$X = \frac{40 \text{ ml}}{10}$$

$$X = 4 \text{ ml}$$

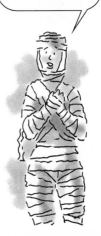

At this rate, I think we'll have a new "mummy" on the unit by the time this problem is finished.

- The flow rate is 4 ml/20 minutes. Because this drug must be delivered by infusion pump, compute the hourly flow rate by multiplying the 20-minute rate by 3:

$$\frac{4 \text{ ml}}{20 \text{ minutes}} \times 3 = 12 \text{ ml/hour}$$

- The hourly flow rate is 12 ml/hour. Lastly, calculate the flow rate to be used after the first 20 minutes, resulting in 3 milliunits/minute (180 milliunits/hour). Having calculated the solution's concentration as 10 milliunits/ml, set up a proportion with the known concentration in one fraction and the increased oxytocin dose and the unknown flow rate in the other fraction:

$$\frac{10 \text{ milliunits}}{1 \text{ ml}} = \frac{180 \text{ milliunits}}{X}$$

- Cross-multiply the fractions:

$$X \times 10 \text{ milliunits} = 1 \text{ ml} \times 180 \text{ milliunits}$$

- Solve for X by dividing both sides of the equation by 10 milliunits and canceling units that appear in both the numerator and denominator:

$$\frac{X \times \cancel{10 \text{ milliunits}}}{\cancel{10 \text{ milliunits}}} = \frac{1 \text{ ml} \times 180 \text{ \cancel{milliunits}}}{10 \text{ \cancel{milliunits}}}$$

$$X = \frac{180 \text{ ml}}{10}$$

$$X = 18 \text{ ml}$$

- After 20 minutes, reset the pump to deliver 18 ml/hour. That's 18 ml/60 minutes, or 0.3 ml/minute. Because there are 10 milliunits/ml, multiply 10 by 0.3 ml/minute to verify that this flow rate does provide 3 milliunits/minute.

Critical care drugs

- Because of the life-threatening nature of patients' conditions, calculations involving critical care drugs need to be performed quickly.
- Many of these drugs are given by I.V. push.
- Generally, drugs are ordered by dosage, which may include mg/minute or mcg/kg/minute.
- Always double-check the vial to make sure that you're giving the right concentration.
- Be prepared when performing calculations to prevent stress.

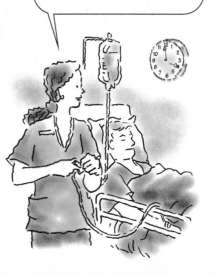

Check your calculations carefully, and double-check the vial to ensure you're giving the right concentration of drug. A mistake could be lethal.

Quick list of critical care meds and measurements

These lists show some of the common critical care drugs and associated units of measure. Memorizing these units of measure helps speed your calculations.

mg/minute
- lidocaine
- phenylephrine
- procainamide

mcg/minute
- epinephrine
- nitroglycerin
- norepinephrine

mcg/kg/minute
- dobutamine
- dopamine
- nitroprusside

Calculating I.V. push dosages

- Calculations of I.V. push drugs are similar to those for I.M. drugs, but administration times may vary.
- If you aren't sure how quickly to administer a drug, look it up in a drug reference.

Learn by example

Your patient is admitted with frequent ventricular arrhythmias. The prescriber orders *procainamide 200 mg q5 min by slow I.V. push until arrhythmias disappear.* If the drug label says the dose strength is 100 mg/ml, how many milliliters of procainamide should you give to the patient every 5 minutes?

- Set up a proportion with the ordered dose and the unknown volume in one fraction and the dose strength in milligrams per milliliter in the other fraction:

Help desk

Stress busters

Here are four hot tips to help reduce your stress level when calculating drugs during an emergency:

✌ Carry a list of all drug-calculation formulas.

✌ Carry a calculator for quick use.

✌ Convert each patient's weight into kilograms, and keep the information at the bedside.

✋ Become familiar with the different critical care drugs given I.V. as well as your unit's medication protocols.

$$\frac{200 \text{ mg}}{X} = \frac{100 \text{ mg}}{1 \text{ ml}}$$

- Cross-multiply the fractions:

$$X \times 100 \text{ mg} = 1 \text{ ml} \times 200 \text{ mg}$$

- Solve for X by dividing each side of the equation by 100 mg and canceling out units that appear in both the numerator and denominator:

$$\frac{X \times \cancel{100 \text{ mg}}}{\cancel{100 \text{ mg}}} = \frac{1 \text{ ml} \times 200 \cancel{\text{ mg}}}{100 \cancel{\text{ mg}}}$$

$$X = \frac{200 \text{ ml}}{100}$$

$$X = 2 \text{ ml}$$

- You should administer 2 ml.

Learn by example

Your patient has a history of rapid atrial fibrillation and takes digoxin at home. When his digoxin level is found to be subtherapeutic, the prescriber orders 0.125 mg I.V. digoxin as a single dose to control his heart rate. The only available digoxin vial contains 0.25 mg/ml. How many milliliters should you give?

I'm sorry... I have to issue you a ticket. Do you have any idea just how fast you were going?

- Set up a proportion with the available solution in one ratio and the ordered dose and the unknown volume in the other ratio:

$$0.25 \text{ mg} : 1 \text{ ml} :: 0.125 \text{ mg} : X$$

- Multiply the means and the extremes:

$$X \times 0.25 \text{ mg} = 1 \text{ ml} \times 0.125 \text{ mg}$$

• Solve for X by diving both sides of the equation by 0.25 mg and canceling units that appear in both the numerator and denominator:

$$\frac{X \times \cancel{0.25\ mg}}{\cancel{0.25\ mg}} = \frac{1\ ml \times 0.125\ \cancel{mg}}{0.25\ \cancel{mg}}$$

$$X = \frac{0.125\ ml}{0.25}$$

$$X = 0.5\ ml$$

• You should administer 0.5 ml of digoxin.

Calculating I.V. flow rates

• You may need to do three different calculations before administering critical care drugs. These include finding the:
  – concentration of the drug in the I.V. solution
  – flow rate required to deliver the desired dose
  – number of micrograms needed, based on the patient's weight in kilograms. (This is needed if the drug is ordered in micrograms per kilogram of body weight per minute.)
• To calculate the drug concentration, use this formula:

Three different calculations, you say? Great! Time enough for a quick yoga stretch before I go back to work.

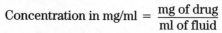

$$\text{Concentration in mg/ml} = \frac{\text{mg of drug}}{\text{ml of fluid}}$$

  – This formula will give you the concentration in mg/ml.
  – If you need to express the concentration in mcg/ml, simply multiply the answer by 1,000.

- To determine the I.V. flow rate per minute, use this formula:

$$\frac{\text{dose/minute}}{X} = \frac{\text{concentration of solution}}{1 \text{ ml of fluid}}$$

- To calculate the hourly flow rate, multiply the ordered dose (in milligrams or micrograms per minute) by 60 minutes.
  - Then use this formula to compute the hourly flow rate:

$$\frac{\text{hourly dose}}{X} = \frac{\text{concentration of solution}}{1 \text{ ml of fluid}}$$

- To determine the dosage in milligrams per kilogram of body weight per minute, take these steps:
  - Determine the concentration of the solution in milligrams per milliliter. To determine the dose in milligrams per hour, multiply the hourly flow rate by the concentration using this formula:

Dose in mg/hour = Hourly flow rate × Concentration

No time for books?

Don't have time to refer to your dosage calculation book in a critical situation? Keep these formulas on a card with your calculator for quick reference. They're foolproof!

- To find out how many micrograms per kilogram per minute your patient is receiving, use this formula:

$$\frac{\text{mg} \times 1{,}000 \div 60 \div \text{kg} \times \text{infusion rate}}{\text{volume of bag}} = \text{mcg/kg/minute}$$

- To find out how many milliliters per hour you should give, use this formula:

$$\frac{\text{weight in kg} \times \text{dose in mcg/kg/minute} \times 60}{\text{concentration in 1 L}} = \text{ml/hour}$$

- Divide the dose per minute by the patient's weight using this formula:

$$mg/kg/minute = \frac{mg/minute}{patient's\ weight\ in\ kilograms}$$

- After performing these calculations, make sure that the drug is being given in a safe and therapeutic range. Compare the amount in milligrams per kilogram per minute to the safe range shown in a drug reference.

Learn by example

Your patient is having frequent runs of ventricular tachycardia that subside after 10 to 12 beats. The prescriber orders 2 g (2,000 mg) lidocaine in 500 ml of dextrose 5% in water (D_5W) to infuse at 2 mg/minute. What's the flow rate in milliliters per minute? In milliliters per hour?

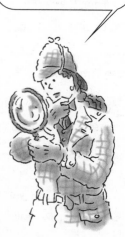

Just what I enjoy— a tantalizing number mystery to solve. The game is afoot!

• Find the solution's concentration by setting up a proportion with the unknown concentration in one fraction and the ordered dose in the other fraction:

$$\frac{X}{1\ ml} = \frac{2,000\ mg}{500\ ml}$$

• Cross-multiply the fractions:

$$X \times 500\ ml = 2,000\ mg \times 1\ ml$$

- Solve for X by dividing each side of the equation by 500 ml and canceling units that appear in both the numerator and denominator:

$$\frac{X \times \cancel{500\ ml}}{\cancel{500\ ml}} = \frac{2{,}000\ mg \times 1\ \cancel{ml}}{500\ \cancel{ml}}$$

$$X = \frac{2{,}000\ mg}{500}$$

$$X = 4\ mg$$

- The solution's concentration is 4 mg/ml. Next, calculate the flow rate per minute needed to deliver the ordered dose of 2 mg/minute. Set up a proportion with the unknown flow rate per minute in one fraction and the solution's concentration in the other fraction:

$$\frac{2\ mg}{X} = \frac{4\ mg}{1\ ml}$$

- Cross-multiply the fractions:

$$X \times 4\ mg = 1\ ml \times 2\ mg$$

- Solve for X by dividing both sides of the equation by 4 mg and canceling units that appear in both the numerator and denominator:

$$\frac{X \times \cancel{4\ mg}}{\cancel{4\ mg}} = \frac{1\ ml \times 2\ \cancel{mg}}{\cancel{4\ mg}}$$

$$X = \frac{2\ ml}{4}$$

$$X = 0.5\ ml$$

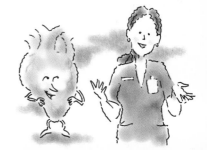

Now that we know how much lidocaine to give per minute, it should be easy figuring out the hourly flow rate.

- The patient should receive 0.5 ml/minute of lidocaine. Lidocaine must be infused on an infusion pump, so calculate the hourly flow rate. Do this by setting up a proportion with the unknown flow rate per hour in one fraction and the flow rate per minute in the other fraction:

$$\frac{X}{60 \text{ minutes}} = \frac{0.5 \text{ ml}}{1 \text{ minute}}$$

- Cross-multiply the fractions:

$$X \times 1 \text{ minute} = 0.5 \text{ ml} \times 60 \text{ minutes}$$

- Solve for X by dividing both sides of the equation by 1 minute and canceling units that appear in both the numerator and denominator:

$$\frac{X \times \cancel{1 \text{ minute}}}{\cancel{1 \text{ minute}}} = \frac{0.5 \text{ ml} \times 60 \cancel{\text{ minutes}}}{\cancel{1 \text{ minute}}}$$

$$X = 30 \text{ ml}$$

- Set the infusion pump to deliver 30 ml/hour.

Learn by example

A 200-lb patient is to receive an I.V. infusion of dobutamine at 10 mcg/kg/minute. The label instructs to check the package insert. There it states to dilute 250 mg of the drug in 50 ml of D_5W. Because the drug vial contains 20 ml of solution, the total to be infused is 70 ml (50 ml of D_5W + 20 ml of solution). How many milliliters of the drug should the patient receive each minute? Each hour?

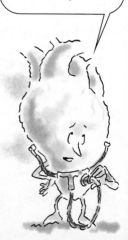

I must concur... a dobutamine infusion at 10 mcg/kg/minute should do the trick nicely.

- First, compute the patient's weight in kilograms. Set up a proportion with the weight in pounds and the unknown weight in kilograms in one fraction, and the number of pounds per kilogram in the other fraction:

$$\frac{200 \text{ lb}}{X} = \frac{2.2 \text{ lb}}{1 \text{ kg}}$$

- Cross-multiply the fractions:

$$X \times 2.2 \text{ lb} = 1 \text{ kg} \times 200 \text{ lb}$$

- Solve for X by dividing both sides of the equation by 2.2 lb and canceling units that appear in both the numerator and denominator:

$$\frac{X \times \cancel{2.2 \text{ lb}}}{\cancel{2.2 \text{ lb}}} = \frac{1 \text{ ml} \times 200 \cancel{\text{ lb}}}{\cancel{2.2 \text{ lb}}}$$

$$X = \frac{200 \text{ kg}}{2.2}$$

$$X = 90.9 \text{ kg}$$

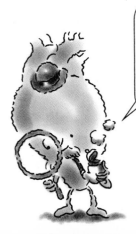

Clever of me to detect the recurring patterns in all these problems... cross-multiplication and solving for X! Why, it's elementary!

- The patient weighs 90.9 kg. Determine the dose in milliliters per minute by setting up a proportion with the patient's weight in kilograms and the unknown dose in micrograms per minute in one fraction and the known dose in micrograms per kilogram in the other fraction:

$$\frac{90.9 \text{ kg}}{X} = \frac{1 \text{ kg}}{10 \text{ mcg/minute}}$$

- Cross-multiply the fractions:

$$X \times 1 \text{ kg} = 10 \text{ mcg/minute} \times 90.9 \text{ kg}$$

- Solve for X by dividing each side of the equation by 1 kg and canceling units that appear in both the numerator and denominator:

$$\frac{X \times \cancel{1 \text{ kg}}}{\cancel{1 \text{ kg}}} = \frac{10 \text{ mcg/minute} \times 90.9 \cancel{\text{ kg}}}{1 \cancel{\text{ kg}}}$$

$$X = 909 \text{ mcg/minute}$$

- The patient should receive 909 mcg of dobutamine every minute, or 0.909 mg every minute. To determine the flow rate in milliliters per minute, set up a proportion using the solution's concentration and solve for X:

$$\frac{0.909 \text{ mg}}{X} = \frac{250 \text{ mg}}{70 \text{ ml}}$$

$$250 \text{ mg} \times X = 0.909 \text{ mg} \times 70 \text{ ml}$$

$$\frac{\cancel{250 \text{ mg}} \times X}{\cancel{250 \text{ mg}}} = \frac{0.909 \text{ mg} \times 70 \text{ ml}}{250 \cancel{\text{ mg}}}$$

$$X = \frac{63.63 \text{ ml}}{250}$$

$$X = 0.25 \text{ ml/minute}$$

- To find the flow rate in milliliters per hour, multiply by 60:

   0.25 ml/minute × 60 minutes/hour = 15 ml/hour

- The patient should receive dobutamine at a rate of 15 ml/hour.

Using special calculations

- Some critical care drugs are prescribed according to the patient's heart rate, blood pressure, or other parameters.
- The prescriber may write a starting dose and a maximum dose to which the drug can be titrated.
- To deliver the correct amount of drug, you must calculate the starting dose and the maximum dose.

Really, we'd all like to hear why you rate your own "special" category.

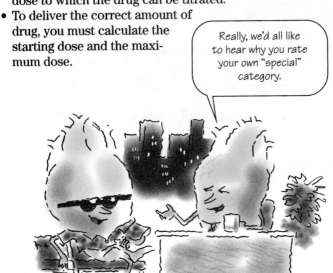

Learn by example

A patient with severe hypertension weighs 85 kg. The order reads *nitroprusside 50 mg in 250 ml of D₅W. Start at 0.5 mcg/kg/minute. Titrate to keep systolic BP less than 170 mm Hg. Maximum dose is 10 mcg/kg/minute.* At what rate should you start the infusion?

- First, find the concentration of the infusion. Start by converting 50 mg to 50,000 mcg:

$$\frac{50,000 \text{ mcg}}{250 \text{ ml}} = 200 \text{ mcg/ml}$$

- Then set up the following equation:

$$X = \frac{85 \text{ kg} \times 0.5 \text{ mcg/kg/minute} \times 60}{200 \text{ mcg/ml}}$$

$$X = 12.75$$

- Rounded off, the starting dose is 13 ml/hour.

The TEST ZONE

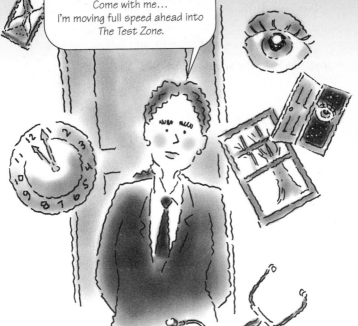
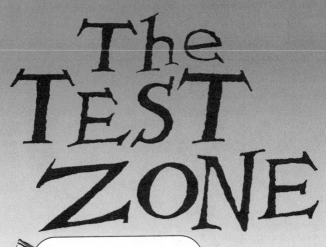

Chapter 1: Math basics

1. Which of the following is an example of a proportion?
   A. 1 : 2 :: 2 : 1
   B. 3 : 6 :: 8 : 4
   C. 5 : 1 :: 10 : 2
   D. 4 : 5 :: 7 : 8
2. The proportion 3 : 2 :: 6 : 4 can be restated in fraction form as:
   A. $^3/_2 = ^6/_4$.
   B. $^2/_3 = ^6/_4$.
   C. $^6/_2 = ^3/_4$.
   D. $^2/_6 = ^4/_3$.
3. A practitioner prescribes 0.75 mg of a drug. The vial that pharmacy sent contains 0.5 mg per ml of solution. How many milliliters of the solution should you administer?
   A. 0.5
   B. 1
   C. 1.5
   D. 2
4. Your patient weighs 187 lb. How much does he weigh in kilograms?
   A. 80
   B. 85
   C. 90
   D. 95

Chapter 2: Measurement systems

5. How many grams are in 5,124 mg?
   A. 0.5124
   B. 5.124
   C. 51.24
   D. 5,124,000
6. How many milliliters of solution are left in a 2-L bag of normal saline solution after you remove 0.75 L, 60 ml, and 230 ml?
   A. 40
   B. 420
   C. 960
   D. 1,635

7. How is the Arabic numeral 670 written in Roman numerals?
    A. CDLXX
    V. DXC
    C. DCLXX
    D. CCCCCCLXV
8. Which drug is commonly ordered in the milliequivalent (mEq) system?
    A. Insulin
    B. Penicillin
    C. Heparin
    D. Potassium

Chapter 3: Recording drug administration

9. In military time, 1:45 p.m. is converted to what number?
    A. 0145
    B. 145
    C. 1345
    D. 2545
10. What's the first thing to do after administering a drug?
    A. Document the time of administration.
    B. Go see the next patient who's waiting.
    C. Answer a phone call from the patient's family member.
    D. Take the patient's vital signs.
11. The abbreviation NKA stands for:
    A. no known adverse reactions.
    B. no known administration.
    C. no known alteration.
    D. no known allergies.
12. The nurse must administer a bolus dose of dextrose 10% in water ($D_{10}W$) to a patient. Another nurse drew up the solution for her and told her that she would leave it at the patient's bedside. When the nurse arrives at the bedside, there are two unmarked syringes. What should the nurse do?
    A. Administer the medication she thinks is the correct one.
    B. Ask the other nurse which syringe is the right one to administer.
    C. Discard both syringes and draw up the $D_{10}W$ again.
    D. Ask the patient which syringe the nurse just set down.

Chapter 4: Oral, topical, and rectal drugs

13. If a patient needs 150 mcg of Synthroid P.O. and the available dose is 50 mcg/tablet, how many tablets should you give?

    A. 2

    B. 3

    C. 4

    D. 5

14. If the prescriber orders 250 mcg of digoxin elixir P.O. stat and the bottle label reads *digoxin 25 mcg per ¹/₂ tsp*, you should give the patient how many milliliters?

    A. 5

    B. 10

    C. 15

    D. 20

15. Which of the following isn't a rule to use when calculating drug dosages?

    A. Question strange answers.

    B. Get out the calculator.

    C. Double-check decimals.

    D. Disregard zeros in your calculation.

16. If a drug label reads *Compazine (prochlorperazine) suppositories 5 mg, GlaxoSmithKline, for rectal use only*, what's the drug's proprietary name?

    A. Compazine

    B. Prochlorperazine

    C. GlaxoSmithKline

    D. Suppositories

Chapter 5: Parenteral drugs

17. Needles used for subQ injections are what size?

    A. ³/₈″ to ⁵/₈″ long and 25G to 27G

    B. ¹/₂″ to ⁵/₈″ long and 23G to 28G

    C. 1″ to 3″ long and 18G to 23G

    D. ³/₄″ long and 22G

18. A percentage solution can be expressed in terms of:

    A. weight/volume and volume/volume.

    B. weight/weight and volume/volume.

    C. weight/weight and strength/volume.

    D. grams/weight and milliliters/volume.

19. Which two types of insulin can be combined together in the same syringe?

A. Lente and ultralente
B. NPH and lispro
C. NPH and regular
D. Regular and Lantus

20. When a diluent is added to a powder for injection, what happens to the fluid volume?

A. It increases.
B. It decreases.
C. It stays the same.
D. It always doubles.

Chapter 6: I.V. infusions

21. For a microdrip set with a drop factor of 60 gtt/ml, the drip rate is:

A. half the hourly flow rate.
B. 10 times greater than the hourly flow rate.
C. the same as the hourly flow rate.
D. four times greater than the hourly flow rate.

22. The prescriber orders 1,000 ml of a drug to infuse over 8 hours at 31 gtt/minute. The set calibration is 15 gtt/ml. After 5 hours, 750 ml have infused, instead of 625 ml. To recalculate the drip rate for the remaining solution, you would:

A. increase the rate to 35 gtt/minute.
B. increase the rate to 40 gtt/minute.
C. slow the rate to 15 gtt/minute.
D. slow the rate to 21 gtt/minute.

23. You need to infuse 2,000 ml of D_5W over 12 hours. What's the flow rate?

A. 167 ml/hour
B. 200 ml/hour
C. 217 ml/hour
D. 230 ml/hour

24. You start a continuous infusion of 100 units of regular insulin in 100 ml of normal saline solution. If the prescribed dose is 9 units/hour, what's the hourly flow rate?

A. 6 units/hour
B. 9 units/hour
C. 12 units/hour
D. 15 units/hour

Chapter 7: Special calculations

25. If the suggested pediatric dosage for a drug is 40 mg/kg/day, the amount to give an infant weighing 7 kg is:
   A. 225 mg.
   B. 250 mg.
   C. 280 mg.
   D. 310 mg.

26. If a patient is 40″ tall, weighs 64 lb, and has a BSA of 0.96 m^2, how much fluid does he require per day?
   A. 140 ml
   B. 1,040 ml
   C. 1,400 ml
   D. 1,440 ml

27. A sudden increase or decrease in the fetal heart rate after drug treatment is considered:
   A. a sign that the infant is about to be delivered.
   B. an adverse reaction to the drug.
   C. a temporary reaction to many obstetric drugs.
   D. a sign indicating that the drug has reached its peak level.

28. A 200-lb patient with minimal urine output has an order to receive dopamine at 5 mcg/kg/minute. The premixed bag of dopamine contains 400 mg in 250 ml of D_5W. How many milliliters of solution containing dopamine will the patient receive each hour?
   A. 17
   B. 18
   C. 19
   D. 20

Answers

Chapter 1: Math basics

1. C. In a proportion, the ratios are equal.

2. A. Make the ratios on both sides into fractions by substituting slashes for colons.

3. C. Substitute X for the amount of solution needed to administer 0.75 mg of the drug, and then set up a proportion with ratios or fractions.

4. B. Use the conversion 2.2 kg = 1 lb. Then set up the equation and do the math:

$$\frac{187 \, \cancel{lb}}{1} \times \frac{1 \, kg}{2.2 \, \cancel{lb}} = \frac{187 \times 1 \, kg}{1 \times 2.2} = \frac{187 \, kg}{2.2} = 85 \, kg$$

Chapter 2: Measurement systems

5. B. Locate *milli* and *gram* on the *Amazing decimal place finder*, page 60, and count the number of places gram is to the left of milli. Then move the decimal point three places to the left.

6. C. Convert all the measurements to milliliters, add the last three numbers to find out how many milliliters were removed from the bag, then subtract this number from the amount of fluid in the bag.

7. C. To convert 670, break it into its component parts (600 and 70), and then translate the parts into Roman numerals (DC and LXX).

8. D. Potassium is measured in milliequivalents.

Chapter 3: Recording drug administration

9. C. To convert a time from 1:00 p.m. to 12 midnight, add 12 to the hour and remove the colon.

10. A. Immediately after administering a drug, document the time of administration in the patient's medication administration record (MAR). This prevents you or another member of the health care team from inadvertently giving the drug again.

11. D. NKA stands for *no known allergies*. Allergy information should always be recorded. If there are no known allergies, document *NKA* in the MAR.

12. C. It's never safe to administer an unlabeled syringe or solution. By discarding both syringes, the nurse eliminates the risk of giving the wrong drug or solution to the patient. Even if the other nurse remembers which syringe had the $D_{10}W$, it's still possible that the syringes became mixed up at the bedside. The appropriate action is to draw up and label a new syringe with $D_{10}W$ to administer to the patient.

Chapter 4: Oral, topical, and rectal drugs

13. B. If 1 tablet provides 50 mcg, divide 150 by 50 to get the answer: 3 tablets.

14. B. First, consult a conversion table to find that 1 tsp equals 5 ml. Then use proportions to solve for X.

15. D. You should always double-check zeros when doing math calculations. A zero in the wrong place can cause a tenfold or greater dosage error.

16. A. The proprietary, or trade, name usually appears first on a drug label— just before or above the generic name.

Chapter 5: Parenteral drugs

17. B. These needles can inject 0.5 to 1 ml subQ.

18. A. Percentage solutions are expressed as weight/volume or volume/ volume. These are the clearest and most common ways to label or describe solutions.

19. C. NPH and regular insulin may be combined together in the same syringe. Draw the regular insulin first and then the NPH.

20. A. When a diluent is added to a powder, the fluid volume increases. That's why the label calls for less diluent than the total volume of the pre- pared solution.

Chapter 6: I.V. infusions

21. C. The drip rate is the same as the hourly flow rate because the number of minutes in an hour—60—is the same as the drop factor.

22. D. To solve this problem, determine the amount of fluid remaining by subtracting 750 ml from 1,000 ml. Convert the time remaining to minutes. Set up the equation using this formula:

$$\frac{\text{Total ml}}{\text{Total minutes}} \times \text{drop factor in gtt/ml} = \text{drip rate in gtt/ml}$$

23. A. To find the answer (167 ml/hour), set up an equation using this formula:

$$\text{Total volume ordered/Number of hours}$$

24. B. Solve this problem by setting up the first fraction with the known solution strength and the second fraction with the desired dose and the unknown volume. Put these fractions into a proportion, cross-multiplying, and then dividing and canceling the units of measure that appear in both the numerator and denominator.

Chapter 7: Special calculations

5. C. To solve this problem, set up a proportion with the suggested dosage in one ratio and the unknown quantity in the other. Multiply the means and extremes and then divide each side of the equation by the value that appears on the X side of the equation. Cancel units that appear in both the numerator and denominator.

6. D. Use the equation for calculating fluid needs based on BSA, inserting the appropriate numbers. Then solve for X.

7. B. Changes in the fetal heart rate may signal an adverse reaction to the drug; therefore, discontinue the drug immediately.

8. A. First, determine the patient's weight in kilograms by dividing his weight in pounds by 2.2 kg (200 ÷ 2.2 = 91 kg). Next, determine the concentration of medication in micrograms by multiplying milligrams by 1,000. Then divide by 250 ml to determine the concentration in 1 ml:

$$\frac{400 \text{ mg}}{250 \text{ ml}} \times \frac{1,000 \text{ mcg}}{1 \text{ mg}} = \frac{400,000 \text{ mcg}}{250 \text{ ml}} = 1,600 \text{ mcg}$$

To find out how many milliliters per hour you should give, use the formula:

weight in kg × dose in mcg/kg/minute × 60 (minutes in 1 hour) ÷ concentration in 1 ml of solution

$$\frac{91 \text{ kg}}{1} \times \frac{5 \text{ mcg}}{\text{kg/minute}} = \frac{455 \text{ mcg}}{1 \text{ minute}}$$

$$\frac{455 \text{ mcg}}{1 \text{ minute}} \times \frac{60 \text{ minute}}{1 \text{ hour}} = \frac{27,300 \text{ mcg}}{1 \text{ hour}}$$

$$\frac{27,300 \text{ mcg/hour}}{1,600 \text{ mcg/ml}} = 17.06 \text{ ml/hour}$$

Lastly, round off the answer to 17 ml/hour.

Scoring

☆☆☆ If you answered 25 to 28 questions correctly, great job! You're in a dimension all by yourself.

☆☆ If you answered 19 to 24 questions correctly, way to go! You're really in the zone.

☆ If you answered fewer than 19 questions correctly, review the chapters and try again. It won't be long until you see the light!

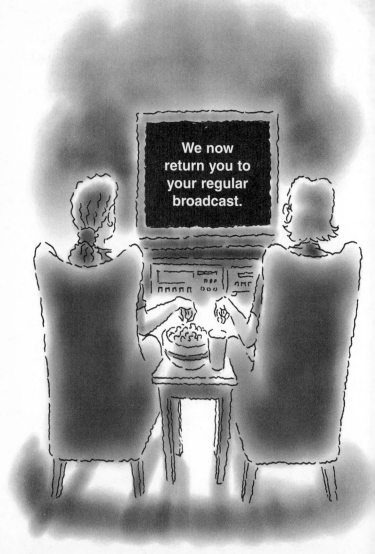

Weight conversion

To convert a patient's weight in pounds to kilograms, divide the number of pounds by 2.2 kg; to convert a patient's weight in kilograms to pounds, multiply the number of kilograms by 2.2 lb.

Pounds	Kilograms
10	4.5
20	9.1
30	13.6
40	18.2
50	22.7
60	27.3
70	31.8
80	36.4
90	40.9
100	45.5
110	50
120	54.5
130	59.1
140	63.6
150	68.2
160	72.7
170	77.3
180	81.8
190	86.4
200	90.9

Temperature conversion

To convert Fahrenheit to Celsius, subtract 32 from the temperature in Fahrenheit and then divide by 1.8; to convert Celsius to Fahrenheit, multiply the temperature in Celsius by 1.8 and then add 32.

$$(F - 32) \div 1.8 = \text{degrees Celsius}$$

$$(C \times 1.8) + 32 = \text{degrees Fahrenheit}$$

Degrees Fahrenheit (°F)	Degrees Celsius (°C)	Degrees Fahrenheit (°F)	Degrees Celsius (°C)
89.6	32	101	38.3
91.4	33	101.2	38.4
93.2	34	101.4	38.6
94.3	34.6	101.8	38.8
95	35	102	38.9
95.4	35.2	102.2	39
96.2	35.7	102.6	39.2
96.8	36	102.8	39.3
97.2	36.2	103	39.4
97.6	36.4	103.2	39.6
98	36.7	103.4	39.7
98.6	37	103.6	39.8
99	37.2	104	40
99.3	37.4	104.4	40.2
99.7	37.6	104.6	40.3
100	37.8	104.8	40.4
100.4	38	105	40.6
100.8	38.2		

Drug therapy conversions

Metric weight

1 kilogram (kg)	= 1,000 grams (g)
1 g	= 1,000 milligrams (mg)
1 mg	= 1,000 micrograms (mcg)
0.6 g	= 600 mg
0.3 g	= 300 mg
0.1 g	= 100 mg
0.06 g	= 60 mg
0.03 g	= 30 mg
0.015 g	= 15 mg
0.001 g	= 1 mg

Metric volume

1 liter (L)	= 1,000 milliliters (ml)
1 ml	= 1,000 microliters (µl)

Household	*Metric*
1 teaspoon (tsp)	= 5 ml
1 tablespoon (T or tbs)	= 15 ml
2 tbs	= 30 ml
8 ounces	= 240 ml
1 pint (pt)	= 473 ml
1 quart (qt)	= 946 ml
1 gallon (gal)	= 3,785 ml

Calculating drip rates

When calculating the flow rate of I.V. solutions, remember that the number of drops required to deliver 1 ml varies with the type of administration set you're using. To calculate the drip rate, you must know the calibration of the drip rate for each specific manufacturer's product. As a quick guide, refer to the chart below. Use this formula to calculate specific drip rates:

$$\frac{\text{volume of infusion (in ml)}}{\text{time of infusion (in minutes)}} \times \text{drip factor (in drops/ml)} = \text{drops/minute}$$

	Ordered volume		
	500 ml/24 hour or 21 ml/hour	1000 ml/24 hour or 42 ml/hour	1000 ml/20 hour or 50 ml/hour
Drops/ml	Drops/minute to infuse		
Macrodrip			
10	4	7	8
15	5	11	13
20	7	14	17
Microdrip			
60	21	42	50

1000 ml/10 hour or 100 ml/hour	1000 ml/8 hour or 125 ml/hour	1000 ml/6 hour or 166 ml/hour
17	21	28
25	31	42
33	42	55
100	125	166

Common calculation formulas

$$\text{Body surface area in m}^2 = \sqrt{\frac{\text{height in cm} - \text{weight in kg}}{3,600}}$$

$$\text{mcg/ml} = \text{mg/ml} \times 1,000$$

$$\text{ml/minute} = \frac{\text{ml/hour}}{60}$$

$$\text{gtt/minute} = \frac{\text{volume in ml to be infused}}{\text{time in minutes}} \times \text{drip factor in gtt/ml}$$

$$\text{mg/minute} = \frac{\text{mg in bag}}{\text{ml in bag}} \times \text{flow rate} \div 60$$

$$\text{mcg/minute} = \frac{\text{mg in bag}}{\text{ml in bag}} \div 0.06 \times \text{flow rate}$$

$$\text{mcg/kg/minute} = \frac{\text{mcg/ml} \times \text{ml/minute}}{\text{weight in kilograms}}$$

Selected references

Brown, M., and Mulholland, J.L. *Drug Calculations: Process & Problems for Clinical Practice*, 7th ed. St. Louis: Mosby–Year Book, Inc., 2004.

Craig, G.P. *Clinical Calculations Made Easy: Solving Problems Using Dimensional Analysis*, 3rd ed. Philadelphia: Lippincott Williams & Wilkins, 2004.

Dosage Calculations Made Incredibly Easy, 3rd ed. Philadelphia: Lippincott Williams & Wilkins, 2005.

Inglebright, J., and Franklin, M. "Managing a New Medication Administration Process," *Journal of Nursing Administration* 35(9):410-13, September 2005.

Warne-Britner, S., et al. "Improving Medication Calculation Skills of Nurses and Nursing Students," *Clinical Nurse Specialist* 19(2):74, March-April 2005.

Husch, M, et al. "Insights from the Sharp End of Intravenous Medication Errors: Implications for Infusion Pump Technology," *Quality and Safety in Healthcare* 14(2):80-86, April 2005.

Macklin, D., et al. *Math for Clinical Practice*. St. Louis: Mosby–Year Book, Inc., 2005.

Nursing2007 Drug Handbook, 27th ed. Philadelphia: Lippincott Williams & Wilkins, 2007.

Ogden, S.J. *Calculation of Drug Dosages*, 7th ed. St. Louis: Mosby–Year Book, Inc., 2003.

Springhouse Nurse's Drug Guide 2007, 8th ed. Philadelphia: Lippincott Williams & Wilkins, 2007.

Taylor, C. *Lippincott's Photo Atlas of Medication Administration*. Philadelphia: Lippincott Williams & Wilkins, 2004.

Index

i refers to an illustration; t refers to a table.

i refers to an illustration; t refers to a table.

i refers to an illustration; t refers to a table.